# YOGA
## RISING

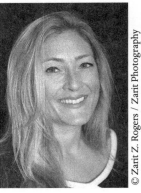

## About the Author

Melanie C. Klein, MA, is a writer, speaker, and professor of Sociology and Women's Studies at Moorpark College in Ventura County, California. Her areas of interest and specialty include media literacy education, body image, and the intersectional analysis of systems of power and privilege. She is the coeditor of *Yoga and Body Image: 25 Personal Stories About Beauty, Bravery & Loving Your Body* (Llewellyn, 2014) with Anna Guest-Jelley, is a contributor in *21st Century Yoga: Culture, Politics and Practice* (Horton & Harvey, 2012), is featured in *Conversations with Modern Yogis* (Shroff, 2014), is a featured writer in *Llewellyn's Complete Book of Mindful Living* (Llewellyn, 2016), and is coeditor of the new anthology *Yoga, the Body and Embodied Social Change: An Intersectional Feminist Analysis* with Dr. Beth Berila and Dr. Chelsea Jackson Roberts (Rowman and Littlefield, 2016). She cofounded the Yoga and Body Image Coalition in 2014. She has been practicing yoga and meditation since 1996 and currently lives in Santa Monica, California.

# MELANIE C. KLEIN

# YOGA RISING

30 Empowering Stories

from Yoga Renegades

for Every Body

Llewellyn Publications
Woodbury, Minnesota

FIRST EDITION
First Printing, 2018

Cover design by Kevin R. Brown
Cover Photograph of Dianne Bondy by Sarit Z Rogers

Llewellyn Publications is a registered trademark of Llewellyn Worldwide Ltd.

**Library of Congress Cataloging-in-Publication Data**
Names: Klein, Melanie, author.
Title: Yoga rising : 30 empowering stories from yoga renegades for every body
   / Melanie C. Klein.
Description: First edition. | Woodbury, Minnesota : Llewellyn Publications,
   2018. | Includes bibliographical references.
Identifiers: LCCN 2017043219 (print) | LCCN 2017048159 (ebook) | ISBN
   9780738755939 (ebook) | ISBN 9780738750828 (alk. paper)
Subjects: LCSH: Yoga—Psychological aspects. | Body image. | Yogis—Biography.
Classification: LCC RA781.67 (ebook) | LCC RA781.67 .K55 2018 (print) | DDC
   613.7/046—dc23
LC record available at https://lccn.loc.gov/2017043219

Llewellyn Publications
A Division of Llewellyn Worldwide Ltd.
2143 Wooddale Drive
Woodbury, MN 55125-2989
www.llewellyn.com

Printed in the United States of America

## Disclaimer

This book is not intended to provide medical advice or to take the place of medical advice and treatment from your personal physician. Readers are advised to consult their doctors or other qualified healthcare professionals regarding the treatment of their medical problems. The publisher and the author recommend common sense when contemplating the practices described in this work.

## Dedication

This book is dedicated to everyone and *every* body who has struggled with self-acceptance, self-doubt, or shame. I see you. Your story matters.

Here's to our personal and collective liberation!

# Contents

# PART FOUR:
## CHALLENGING EXCLUSIVITY AND CREATING SPACE - 181

# PART FIVE:
## IGNITING YOUR INNER YOGA RENEGADE - 229

# FOREWORD

## *by Dianne Bondy*

Despite decades of personal practice, as a person of color I've often felt like yoga practice was not for me. More than four years ago I was compelled to share my experience in the groundbreaking anthology *Yoga and Body Image: 25 Personal Stories About Beauty, Bravery & Loving Your Body.* My hope was that I might connect with yoga practitioners (or those considering a yoga practice) who were struggling with similar feelings of inadequacy, shame, and fear, as well as those who felt excluded from the practice and/or those not represented in yoga media. Frankly, this is most of us.

As the Yoga and Body Image Coalition—an organization that works tirelessly to advocate for accessible, body positive yoga—and I constantly proclaim, "Representation matters." This representation includes the stories that are told, the images that are created, and the work that is shared. Representation matters because diversity is what gives us all a broader and more well-rounded perspective on what it means to be alive and human, as well as how we can coexist together and reach our fullest potential individually and collectively. It matters because together we rise. Together we uplift one another, as well as society as a whole.

*Yoga and Body Image*, the first book in this important series of personal narratives, was offered as a healing balm filled with inspiring stories about lives transformed by mindfulness practices, specifically yoga practice in all its diverse forms. It provided a glimpse into the lives and experiences of yoga practitioners that exist outside the conventional perspectives of what a yogi looks like, challenged the notion of a "yoga body," and expanded our definition of what "yoga" is while inviting readers to connect, become introspective, and step on the mat.

The newest celebration of our yoga stories, *Yoga Rising: 30 Empowering Stories from Yoga Renegades for Every Body,* continues that mission, with the intention and purpose to share the diverse voices and experiences in our collective struggle for understanding, compassion, healing, and equity. It explores the power of the human spirit and the strength of community.

*Yoga Rising* celebrates the spirit of connection through our collective storytelling. Our stories intersect at a common path, revealing that we all belong on the mat because we are all vulnerable, we are all capable and worthy, and we all deserve to be witnessed and valued. It is this connection that reminds us that we are one. We can come to recognize that our differences are meant to be celebrated as a part of our collective consciousness. Each story in this collection (and each of our own personal experiences) represents the larger landscape of what inclusion looks like, from the mat to the studio to representation in media.

Being a yoga renegade means we resist and, more importantly, we persist in challenging and changing the limited narrative of who does yoga and *#whatayogilookslike*[1] is represented by the dominant culture— and far beyond the practice, culture, and business of yoga into the culture at large. I believe there is a renegade in all of us, a renegade dedicated to truth, justice, and equality in all forms. It is through the collective spirit of rebellion illustrated in the stories throughout this book that allow us to move beyond the limited, one-dimensional, and exclusive representations of beauty, health, worth, and value that flood the culture. The stories in this book demonstrate to the world that we are all

1. *#whatayogilookslike* is the Yoga and Body Image Coalition's social media hashtag used to unite body-positive yoga practitioners around the world.

worthy and valuable as we are. It is our collective mantra that we all belong here; all bodies are welcome; all beings are welcome; come and be at peace in and with this practice, free of shame and judgment.

I'm honored to be part of a series of books that have laid the groundwork in changing the mainstream narrative of yoga as merely a function of corporate standards of "beauty" and "fitness." Throughout, this book illustrates how yoga may be used as a tool for empowerment, self-love, and raising our collective consciousness. Throughout, we see firsthand that bodies of every race and ethnicity, gender identity and sexual orientation, age, social class, and levels of abilities can practice alongside each other. In the end, we discover that all our stories carry a common sutra, or thread, of bravery, beauty, and self-awareness.

We are living in a uniquely powerful time, one in which the world is watching as body-positivity and yoga continues to grow in interest and influence. As these ideas continue to rise, more and more people are invited to come to the mat, share their practice and their stories, as well as affirm and reaffirm that this practice has a sacred place for them.

*Yoga Rising* inspires us to share our practice and our stories in the ways that connect with us, both as individuals and as a community. Together we rise, and together we understand that the world has room for all of us. Yoga can lift our hearts, our souls, and our humanity. Yoga has the power to change our perspective, and by changing our point of view, we can change the world. May we be rebellious in our acts of inclusion and love.

—Dianne Bondy, June 2017
Tecumseh, Ontario, Canada

# INTRODUCTION

*Choosing love, we also choose to live
in community, and that means we do not
have to change by ourselves.*
*—bell hooks*

The conversation on the intersection of yoga and body image has experienced a tremendous growth spurt over the last three to four years. Witnessing and participating in the dynamic evolution of this conversation has filled me with great delight and joy. Not only has there been an increase in the number of people and organizations advocating yoga as a tool to promote the development of self-acceptance and a healthy body image but the depth of conversation has been heartening.

Spouting affirmations of body-positivity and "self-love" can fall flat when they aren't supported with the depth and breadth of inquiry required to not only encourage individuals to cultivate an inner paradigm shift but also create large scale cultural change. What has thrilled me the most is how profoundly the dialogue on yoga and body image has developed, replete with all its complexities and nuances. Rather than shying away from simple answers, the collective work of innumerable individuals and organizations across North America and many other parts of the world has exposed and challenged the *structures* and *systems* that promote body dissatisfaction as a personal trouble rather than a larger public issue that spans the spectrum of human experience (not to mention reaps profits from this discontent and desire to "fix" oneself).

As feminists decried long ago, "the personal is political." Both yoga and body image (as well as converging issues as in "yoga and body image"), were long considered as apolitical. Yoga has often been viewed as empty navel gazing or a narcissistic preoccupation with self while body image issues have often been defined as "feminism lite." It has been an important step forward to see the lens of "the personal is political" increasingly applied to these analysis of both yoga and body image (and, "yoga and body image"). Both yoga and the formation of and influence on our body image are not removed from the larger social, political, and economic context that we all exist within. In fact, while individuals create, re-create, and exist within those systems, issues of oppression and exclusivity are rooted within the systems, not the individuals. For example, feminism is often (mis)represented as anti-male when it is actually anti-patriarchy. Recognizing this fact and using it as a new (and increasingly mainstream) way to understand and talk about yoga and body image is nothing short of radical and inspiring.

When I met Anna Guest-Jelley, founder of Curvy Yoga and my co-editor on *Yoga and Body Image: 25 Personal Stories About Beauty, Bravery & Loving Your Body*, in 2010, the yoga blogosphere was just beginning to unfold. Despite individual work and the work some were doing with their students, there wasn't a lot of critical public dialogue around the issues of body image, diversity, inclusivity, and the ways in which a yoga practice can support deep healing from systematic oppression (or, conversely, the ways in which the dominant "yoga culture" often mirrors and exacerbates the cacophony of toxic messaging disseminated by the culture at large). In fact, the few "yoga renegades" who were publicly driving these often confronting and challenging conversations to the foreground in online yoga spaces experienced serious pushback and resistance. It was not uncommon to have this attempt at critical dialogue met with dismissive and condescending remarks as well as claims that those who discussed, confronted, and called out racism, sexism, homophobia, ableism, classism, and ageism in yoga spaces were "negative" and "unyogic." Apparently, you were a "hater" or "jealous" of fill-in-the-blank if you were compelled to dive into deep waters rather than keep your head in the clouds. In fact, in too many cases, the person would be met with exactly the kind of fill-in-the-ism they were exposing and challenging. It was often a frustrating, if not disappointing and painful, experience.

## The Unfolding (R)evolution

We've come a long way. Eight years later, public dialogue on the ways in which body image intersects with race and ethnicity, sexual orientation, gender identity, dis/ability, class and socioeconomic status, age, size, as well as capitalism and culture not only continue to grow but also represent an emergent trend both in yoga spaces and the larger culture beyond the mat and the meditation cushion. To sidestep and ignore these conversations has rendered many publications, companies, and individuals as out of touch and, in some cases, irrelevant (if not obsolete). Spiritual practice and social justice are no longer seen as unrelated or counterintuitive. In fact, more and more individuals and organizations are clearly demonstrating the inevitable ways in which they are woven together.

Despite the resistance and pushback, the conversation has not dimmed. In fact, it has grown in intensity and depth. We've witnessed tangible results across the board—in teaching practices; shifts in studio offerings; the use of language; content creation; collaborative opportunities; and both live and digital conferences, programs, and teacher training offerings that center to name a few. Individuals often feel powerless to create change, but the changes listed here shine an unmistakable light on the power of the individual as part of a larger wave of collective community action.

While we've witnessed a profound shift in the tide, a continued (and deepened) discussion on the intersection of yoga and body image is more relevant than ever. We've made change happen, but the potential healing balm of yoga and meditation is still not accessible to all. Countless blocks continue to exist, thereby barring the possibility of personal and collective liberation for too many—and that's what we're after in the end, our ability to emancipate ourselves from oppressive thoughts, habits, and systems. Just as I benefit from my own sense of increased peace and increased self-worth, I benefit from yours.

While the stereotype of the "yoga body" and misconceptions about who practices yoga (no, you don't have to be white, thin, able-bodied, and bendy) and what yoga practice is (no, it's not a gymnastics course or training for the circus) have been challenged and yoga media has seen increased diversification from magazine covers to feature stories and advertisements, this is still not the norm in yoga culture or the culture at large. In fact, too often diversified content or features on "diversity" are presented as editorial content that exists immediately next to advertisements and media content that undermines these efforts at inclusivity. That is to say, "diversity" is slipped in here and there and the rest of what we see is "business as usual." Until diverse representation is a norm, meaning it becomes the established and unquestioned standard, the conversation and our work is not complete. Because what is desired is the possibility for everyone and every *body* to have access to the practice, benefit from its results, and cultivate self-acceptance and, possibly, full-blown self-love.

## Storytelling as a Revolutionary Act of Love

There is power in storytelling proclaiming our truth, especially as the culture engine continues to grind out misrepresentations and tired stereotypes. The contributors in this book speak their authentic truth. In proclaiming our own truth, no matter how scary or vulnerable it may be, we also provide the opportunity for others to see themselves reflected in our story and, perhaps, provide the courage for them to proclaim their own.

This book became necessary for many reasons. Because the work of demanding and creating inclusivity and equity is far from over. Because a culture that encourages and nurtures self-acceptance, self-love, and body-positivity is still far from the norm. Because the myth of the "yoga body" is still the number one representation in yoga media. Because there are so many brave and inspiring stories to share. Because we can never learn enough about ourselves and the diverse realities of others. For all those reasons (and more), it was clear from the get-go that *Yoga and Body Image: 25 Personal Stories About Beauty, Bravery & Loving Your Body* would only be the first attempt of several to showcase, uplift, and ignite the many stories that need to be shared.

The contributors in *Yoga Rising* have come from all walks of life and backgrounds. Some of them I have known personally either as friends, colleagues, or allies, and in some cases, all of the above. I have met some online by following their work; others I've met in person through shared communities. Some of the contributors wrote to me and shared the ways in which the first book moved them and revealed their unique experiences before I extended an invitation to write for this book. Others were referred to me. There are still others I could not include!

Hopefully, you'll see yourself reflected in at least one, if not a few, of the narratives contained herein. But, here's the *real* gift in reading the lived experiences of others: speaking our truth also creates the unique opportunity for us to identify with those experiences that are *different* from our own. And, maybe (hopefully!), someone else's narrative will make us uncomfortable or angry and push us to our current edge. I mean, we're exploring things that may be painful—not only the -isms as systems of structured inequality, but the pain, shame, and blame that accompany them. Inevitably, these stories will push us out of our comfort zone and challenge our own beliefs and experiences. Can we breathe, listen, and absorb without rushing to challenge the author's experience or truth? Can we honor and respect their truth without feeling like their experience undercuts or invalidates our own? Can we recognize each person's process as uniquely their own, often situated at different points in the progression of healing? Is it possible that our own process is bolstered by theirs, even if we can't recognize it as such in the moment we may be confronted?

Because, in the end, we benefit from this revolutionary act of truth telling. As we connect with our innermost self as well as others through personal narratives and storytelling, our capacity for empathy, compassion, and love grows exponentially—love in every capacity. bell hooks describes love as a radical act of liberation.[1] Consider this book as a collection of love songs designed to support your personal journey toward self-acceptance and, possibly in time, self-love while providing you with the support and care from a community dedicated to that same end. Together we can heal, uplift, and grow toward not only the possibility that we may all see ourselves as enough but the possibility of collective healing and liberation.

## A Call to Move Inward and Outward

To help ignite your own "yoga renegade" and become an agent of change, I've included questions to consider and direct calls to action at the end of each section of this book. No doubt the stories in this collection will bring up lots of feelings and thoughts. Sometimes it's helpful to have some extra support and guidance in consciously examining our own experiences. The questions to consider are designed to help you ponder the ideas presented in the book in a new, different, or deeper way. The calls to action are small, simple (but not necessarily "easy") ways you can begin to move your enthusiasm, energy, emotions, and resolve out into the world in a way that is productive, positive, and beneficial to you and everyone you may have contact with both in person and through social media.

By first moving consciously inward and then outward, we can go out into the world with mindfulness, compassion, and newfound clarity to make shift happen. It doesn't matter how large or small the actions you may take, it's the movement outward into the world that matters and will create a ripple effect. No matter how you are able to or moved to take action, it's the engaged and thoughtful intention to *do* that fuels the fire and helps build on the work of others. Because we're in this together.

Here's to connecting to the truth in our hearts and then connecting to the truth in the hearts of others. May we come together and recognize and support our collective growth.

---

1. bell hooks, *All About Love: New Visions* (New York: William Morrow, 2000).

# PART ONE

## *Yoga, Body Image, and Self-Worth*

You are about to embark on the many essays that have come together in a united voice and message for hope and change. In this first section, you will see that this book starts by picking up the dominant thread presented in *Yoga and Body Image*. Yoga can serve as an instrumental tool in developing care and compassion for ourselves while bolstering self-esteem. And who can't use a bit of that kind of healing remedy?

Both professionally and personally, Lisa Diers (author of the first essay you will soon read) reminds us that learning to love ourselves is possible, even if it may not be realistic at all times. Rather, she encourages readers to come to a place of acceptance with a focus on feeling and function rather than form.

Pia Guerrero shares the intimate intersection of her mother's own leaning toward lifelong dieting with her personal focus on being "perfect" in every sense of the word. Guerrero's diagnosis with Lupus culminated in deep disdain for her body as well as bouts of disordered eating. Upon discovering yoga and recognizing it as a spiritual practice, she created space to allow compassion and forgiveness into her life, attributes and qualities she not only extended to others but to herself.

The pursuit of perfection is an all too common theme when discussing negative body image, disordered eating, and eating disorders. In fact, for Robyn Baker the roots of perfection and her desire for her parents' praise and recognition manifested in her becoming "a ghost of a girl," disappearing pound by pound until she nearly died. Baker eventually discovered how to breathe into "imperfection."

Accompanying notions of perfection is the inner critic, nagging and unforgiving. Through her professional expertise and her own lived experience, Melissa Mercedes focuses on how we can respond to the inner critic and, eventually, bid it farewell.

Jivana Heyman shares the depths of his own despair, the self-hatred stemming from the recognition that he was attracted to men at a time when being gay was not even remotely acceptable. Yoga signaled a single moment of profound transformation in his relationship with self, one that led to self-acceptance and deep service to his community.

Jenny Copeland rounds out the first section with a vulnerable and beautiful essay on the dangers of living small. Yoga offered her the ability to come to her body, be still and listen. And with patience and practice, allow her to take her power back and see herself as a whole being, one worthy and valuable.

Yoga is an opportunity for us all to come home to our full and complete selves. Welcome!

# REDISCOVER, RECONNECT, AND REPAIR: A LIFELONG COMMITMENT

*Lisa Diers*

Your relationship to your body is the longest relationship you'll ever have. To expect to be "in love" with it all the time is unrealistic. To be at war with it is not the answer either. But can you appreciate, respect, and love your body even if you are not always "in love" with how it looks, feels, or functions? Can this be done at a time of everyday body objectification via all mediums of media that use emotionally clever, manipulative, and disempowering messages aimed at our insecurities, perceived shortcomings, and ailments, creating a void for which only "blank" product, procedure, or belief system can fill? In the era of image-dominant forms of expression and communication, with good intentions or otherwise, can you develop a noncompetitive relationship to your body rooted in camaraderie and friendship? Yes, you can.

For more than ten years, I have worked exclusively in eating disorder treatment as both a dietitian nutritionist and a yoga instructor at The Emily Program. I understand both personally and professionally the food and body challenges so many people face. My hope is that sharing some of my experiences and thoughts with you proves helpful and hopeful on your journey toward developing a deeper understanding of and curiosity toward the relationship you have with your body—even in a world that seemingly has the cards stacked against you. I hope that by reading this essay (and the others in this book), the ideas for social change and ways to create a body-positive environment wherever you go spark a fire within you. My greatest hope is that all people can begin to see past the external layer of the body and into the most beautiful part of a person—their soul.

## My Body: A Storied Relationship

Every*BODY* has a story to tell. You may very likely relate to similar experiences of hurt, violation, worry, and mistrust, with the body taking the brunt of the suffering. For many, an instinctual coping mechanism for pain and intense emotions is to find some sense of control and numbing of feelings through food and the powerful distraction of being preoccupied with changing one's body. For all, the body holds experiences. Until we can begin to reconnect to, rediscover, and repair those experiences, we will not know peace.

My body has been an amazing follower of my critical mind from the young age of eight years old. At various times in my life, I have defied my natural weight by being underweight, overweight, fit, and unfit. I have both hated and loved my body at all of these sizes. I know what it feels like to be judged for being on both ends of the weight and appearance spectrum and also in a healthy place and still be judged. I also know what if feels like to arrive at the place of having a deeply rooted, authentic, honest, and respectful relationship with my body. Over its life span, my body has been the armor that has protected me. It has also received a few significant blows that cracked its protective layer. And through it all—through all the times I swore I'd never measure up or I thought the struggle, pain, and heartache would never end—I blamed myself and was convinced that my body was the problem and that by changing it I would find the solutions. Through it all, my body stood by me, waiting patiently, until I figured it out. Its unwavering love and wisdom eventually stood the test of time and shone through. I have a deep love and respect for my body that has been built by the experiences we have lived through together. I accept my body's forms and iterations, see the important purposes for each, and use that wisdom to navigate my work with others and my future.

## Creating an Image

My relationship to my body is like any other deeply committed relationship; it's had a complicated history! Some memories I have of women I looked up to often include their latest diet, negative body comments, and the need to constantly lose weight. These experiences played a role in shaping my self-perception. How could women I thought the world of think of themselves in this way? If something was wrong with their bodies, then there certainly must be something wrong with mine.

At that time, people were mostly unaware of how damaging these appearance-focused comments or unhealthy forms of weight manipulations were on impressionistic minds. The women of that era were without the level of understanding and knowledge of theses struggles that we have today. *Negative body image* wasn't even a known phrase. *Eating disorder*? What was that? We have more knowledge than ever and I couldn't be more proud to be a part of an organization committed to destigmatizing these so very common struggles. These early experiences and the one's that followed connected me with a passion within. At the age of twelve, I realized I wanted to help other people feel better about themselves. As I began to find my own inner peace, that fiery passion to help others grew stronger. As I mended my own relationship to my body, I deeply wanted others to see there was so much more to life than what you did or didn't eat in a day or the number on the scale. It was so much better to be at peace!

I also wanted people to consider that their negative food- and appearance-focused actions and thoughts may be just as dangerous as an addiction to smoking. With that consideration, certainly negative and disordered comments made around others were just as damaging as secondhand smoke.

My mission for change began in college by making a vow to love myself first and to practice compassion toward myself and others. I moved away from body- and appearance-focused comments. I began to question everything I saw in all forms of media and quickly realized how body-centered approaches to marketing were not only skewing self-perception, but also were sneaky attempts to create or validate insecurities as an attempt to sell the solution. I saw myself for who I really was, and I wanted others to see that for themselves. I also became bored by what I felt were trivial conversations surrounding diets, weight, exercise, and appearance. I was irritated that so many women around me overshadowed their greatness with food and body judgments. I saw the waste in it and had enough. Although the journey to body acceptance was a very difficult one, for me, it is what needed to happen so I could both relate to others and help do my part to stop the cycle. I have no anger or resentment toward those times in my life. Although I wouldn't wish them on anyone, those challenging times shaped my future and who I am today.

## How Yoga Discovered Me: Practice Makes Progress

In my twenties, while working in a suburban hospital outside of Minneapolis, my manager asked the dietitians to partner up on a topic they were unfamiliar with, study it, and present it during the next staff meeting. One of my colleagues suggested yoga. I hadn't heard of yoga before and, being a lover of learning, I figured why not?! We did our research and I was never more confused and curious about something in my life!

It wasn't until I took my first "official" yoga class two years later that I began to understand yoga. I took a community class, looking for a way to de-stress and calm down. It was one of the most familiar and natural things I had experienced. For the first time since I could remember, I felt complete, relaxed, and at peace. I remember being so engaged during class and leaving with this thought: *I wonder if I could become a teacher some day.* Four years later, I did.

Since that time, yoga has helped me see that my body holds a wisdom of its own. It is a part of me that can powerfully reflect change, circumstances, or emotions that are challenging to verbally express. Through yoga, I have learned to give my body a voice and try to understand the language it speaks with curiosity and compassion.

Our bodies are such amazing followers of our minds—doing what it commands. When it cannot perform in the way we would like, our body tolerates, in a saintlike way, the verbal and physical abuse we subject it to for not meeting our expectations. I have much remorse for how I treated my body years ago—I truly believe the body is not to blame. Even in times of terminal illness or tragedy, bodies don't fail. Bodies protect, defend, and do their best to adapt to the situation at hand.

My yoga practice and my instruction have changed the way I talk to and about my body. Now, this doesn't mean that I don't get self-conscious at times. Of course I do! But with these thoughts, I try to *"Catch it. Challenge it and change it."* I can see the emotion with my wise mind and have a conscious choice of action, reaction, or non-reaction. My practice has most definitely taught me that. It has taught me how to separate myself from my emotions. To notice where my mind goes when I become uncomfortable in my body or otherwise, and to know that I do not have to react to those emotions. Through the practice of yoga, I have seen that all emotions have a life cycle, just like everything else. There is a beginning, a middle, and an end. I can invite my breath to calm my mind, for one example, and see the emotional cycle end without reacting to it in a negative way. My body deserves better.

Also, when I practice yoga, my body gets a turn to speak. When I don't do yoga or when I don't check in with my body's messages on a regular basis, it gets fed up and demands to be heard in ways that are often frustrating or inconvenient. The body is powerful, so I would much rather make sure it has a regular chance to "speak"!

## Lessons I Have Learned on the Mat

**Lesson 1:** The body can serve as a great and important communicator. Listen to what it has to tell you. Be curious. Not furious.

**Lesson 2:** We all have a body image—a perception of ourselves. I believe the image is on a spectrum and capping the ends of this body image spectrum are the feelings "elation" and "devastation"—those are extremes. You can live in the middle and visit the extremes from time to time and realize it is not a static relationship. Try not to react to it, but learn from it. Listen to it.

**Lesson 3:** Yoga postures are only one small part of yoga. Asana is about function and not about form. Let go of what it looks like, lean in to how it feels, and be open to where it takes you.

**Lesson 4:** Face your fears. If anything scares me, I am curious about that. In yoga, it often plays out in resistance. In those instances, finding my foundational and safe pose is often helpful. Next, to the degree it feels right, I follow my body's lead and oscillate toward instability. When I notice emotional or physical signs of instability on the brink of overwhelm, I breathe to see if that shifts anything. When needed, I move toward stability. This is yoga. Listening to your body, seeing past the fears in your mind to the freedom on the other side. It's knowing life is a process, not perfection. Yoga cannot be the same from pose to pose because the body is never exactly the same from moment to moment.

**Lesson 5:** Discover your poses and yogic techniques. Although no yoga practice or moment is the same, there can be poses that are your safe and stable poses for exploration and reconnection. Familiarity invites safety. Safety invites opportunity to explore. Exploration invites transformation.

**Lesson 6:** Trust and be true to yourself. At the end of the day you have to answer to yourself. Believe in yourself. You hold the answers you need. You are unlimited.

As we have so many visuals available to us, just remember, yoga is not about what it looks like. Yoga is about how it feels to you. That is what is most important. I have recovered and repaired my relationship to food and my body to 100 percent love for who I am. This repair work happened in a variety of ways and yoga sealed it in. It helps me remember what life is really all about.

## Weaving the Tapestry of Change

At the age of twelve, I knew I wanted to do something meaningful in life and it would involve helping others. That has never wavered. One of the best lessons my parents instilled in me early on in life was that one of the most important things a person can do to create change is to start from the change that needs to happen within. From there on, I was regularly reminded and encouraged by them to find and live in my truth, to trust my instincts, stay strong, be kind, remain open and curious, and stand up for what I believe in, no matter what anyone else says. These messages have remained powerful ones throughout my life, helping to direct and steer me wherever the road leads. I believe that all of us have the ability to connect to our inner strengths in this way. Surround yourself with people who support you.

Once I fully understood what negative body image and disordered eating was, how damaging it was to the gift of life, and that I was on the path to freedom, I was on a mission to turn something painful into something positive. I knew this was what I was meant to do.

My Body Positive Social Change Campaign began almost twenty years ago! My life's work chose me, and I trusted the process. Helping people recover from negative body image and disordered eating was my "career goal" as a dietitian. At that time, there were two places in Minnesota to do this work. I knew of one and then saw The Emily Program had a job opening. I put my entire heart and soul in that application and was beyond thrilled when I was scheduled for an interview. As I waited in the lobby for my first interview to begin, I couldn't believe how comfortable and inviting this clinic was. I knew I had come to the right place. After my interview with Dirk Miller, our founder, I left knowing where I needed to be. I walked down the hall to the restroom and did a happy dance chock-full of fist pumps! I wasn't sure what kind of impression I had made or if I would make it to the next round of interviews, but I knew I had never felt more connected to a program, its mission, and the deep sense that this job was for me!

More than ten years later, I have been fully supported in development of our yoga program and honored to be a part of our client's healing journey in this way. Our clients call our approach to yoga "Emily Program Yoga," and our amazing staff of more than twenty registered teachers are specially trained in "Emily Program Approach" to eating disorder –sensitive yoga taught in all locations, levels of care, and groups nationwide. We offer more than fifty yoga classes a week to our clients of all types of disordered eating, body shapes, sizes, abilities, ages, experiences, activity level, trauma experiences, gender, anxiety, depression, race, sexual orientation, you name it. Eating disorders do not discriminate and neither does yoga.

With the utmost care for our clients, we also collaborate with the University of Minnesota to conduct research on how yoga actually helps with body image and disordered eating. We are committed to exploring the role yoga can play in prevention as well as treatment. As we begin our third research study in this area, I am proud of what our clients have taught me, the ideas formed, and the research that can happen to help better understand yoga's role in making a difference in how people experience their relationship to their bodies.

Although we love how safe and supported our clients feel in The Emily Program yoga classes, what concerns me is the weekly requests from our clients for studios that teach like we do at The Emily Program. Regularly I hear from clients how they enjoy the yoga we offer at TEP, but they cannot find yoga like this anywhere else. In my mind, this must change, as yoga instructors have a responsibility to teach yoga that is accessible to all.

Well, my next mission is to change that! With the support of The Emily Program Foundation, my team and I are able to conduct yoga instructor and professional trainings on creating body-positive and eating disorder–sensitive yoga classes and studio environments. Through our blog posts, YouTube videos, writing, teaching, and speaking about positive and realistic body image and "Emily Program Yoga," we can hopefully make a difference in helping repair body-mind relationships. To me, beauty is confidence, kindness, and compassion. That's it. It's all internal and not external. The internal shines through and projects upon the external. With time, this will show externally and add to the body-positive change so desperately needed in our culture.

Yoga is a tool and a versatile one for many to have in the recovery toolbox. Remember, your yoga journey is unique to you. As you begin your campaign to change from within, know you are taking the most important step in changing how our culture views the human body. Slow down, listen, be patient, be compassionate and kind to yourself. You are the only YOU you'll ever have.

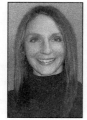

Lisa Diers, RDN, LD, E-RYT, is director of nutrition and yoga program manager at The Emily Program. She is passionate about the healing power that nutrition and yoga provide to those struggling with disordered eating and negative body image. Lisa has led numerous yoga and eating disorder research studies, conducts professional teacher trainings on body image and eating disorder–sensitive yoga, leads The Emily Program yoga blog and YouTube videos, as well as authored book chapters and articles on the these topics.

Author photo by Nancy Linden.

# PERFECTIONISM AND MY PATHWAY TO YOGA

## Pia Guerrero

"One more bite," my mom encouraged me most nights at the dinner table. "Okay ... Take a bite for every year that you are old. One—two—three—four ... Six. Good! You're all finished." She'd smile as she pulled the last forkful of dinner out of my mouth. By seven years old, I was an active and outgoing kid. I climbed trees, talked to strangers, skinned my knees, and won first prize at the bubble gum–eating contest. I was good at pretty much everything. Except eating. Whether it was because of the smell of my mom's liver and onion recipe or because it didn't take much to fuel my small size, I didn't really eat very much as a child.

And why would I? For most of my life, my mom was on a diet, sending me the message loud and clear that food and the enjoyment of it were bad. I also learned that my mom's body was a battlefield, and fat was the enemy—planting the seeds for how I would view my own body one day. As a kid, I knew more about the diet doctors Atkins, Pritikin, and Tarnower than I did about the presidents of the United States. But I did look forward to when my mom would diet. I didn't mind the bland dinners of meat slabs and unseasoned vegetables. I cherished this time together, for it was the closest thing to a family dinner we would have.

## The Sober Life

As a recovering alcoholic, my mom's nights were often filled with AA meetings. So, dinner was never treated as an event to savor or share. Instead, it was something to get through before the babysitter came over. Some nights, Mom was too busy to join us for dinner. The minute she walked in the door from work, she served dinner, rushed through a bunch of chores, and then left for a meeting.

My mom said she met God and sobriety early one morning after she woke up on the hardwood floor, completely oblivious to how she got there, her knees bleeding, and myself asleep in bed. She eventually joined the Self-Realization Fellowship in the late seventies as part of her spiritual journey that came with not drinking. Soon she began studying the teachings of Paramahansa Yogananda, her guru and the founder of SRF, and she committed completely to church activities, chanting, meditation, and yoga. I was in second grade when I was taught how to meditate. More accurately, I tried my best to sit still and fix my closed eyes into the spot between my eyebrows. I absolutely loved contorting my little body into different yoga positions, and, like my mom, I soon began to eat healthy, bland food that my uncle from Utah jokingly called, "nuts and twigs." We made our own peanut butter and had a champion juicer on the counter. "Drink your food and eat your drink," my mom often chirped, quoting her guru.

While my sister and I were ambivalent about joining SRF, we did love how we suddenly were doing things as a family. Mom was no longer rushing through our lives and was grounded and happy. She could finally sit still and be present. At the same time, I didn't understand concepts like karma and reincarnation or who this dead guru guy was or why there were pictures of him hanging around the house. It all felt a little strange, and a sense of alienation was one that lingered through much of my life.

## Sickness and Objectification

I began dancing ballet very seriously. I went to a college-prep school that told us seventh graders to keep up with our academic performance, because it would go on our "permanent record," instilling in me a tremendous fear of failure. We had three-hour finals in every subject, including Latin. This, combined with the perfectionism that came with being the child of an alcoholic and being entrenched in strident ballet school culture every day, made me begin to deteriorate emotionally and physically. I was riddled with anxiety around my future. *Could I keep up? Was I smart enough? Hell ... was I even smart?*

The summer after eighth grade, I was diagnosed with Lupus. Type A personalities are at a higher risk of developing the disease. And that was when my relationship with my body changed. My strong, little, thin body was no longer a fun vehicle for play and self-expression. My knees and hands became blown-up, creaky, arthritic hinges, making it impossible to dance. I was in pain and out of breath all the time. With the Lupus came a diagnosis of fibromyalgia, and I officially became a "sick person." I was put on massive doses of cortisone, with side effects that included a dramatic redistribution of fat and retention of a lot of water. A "buffalo hump," as the doctors called it, began accumulating behind my neck. I grew a "moon face" and a double chin. My tummy bloated out and the drug wasted away my arms and legs.

I began to hate my body—how it looked and the fact that it could no longer move the way it once had, thanks to pain and side effects of the medicine. I had to limit foods as a way to not tax my failing kidneys that the Lupus had been attacking. As a result, I soon developed an episode of disordered eating. In addition to the progression of the disease, I felt I could somehow control the drug-induced double chin, the buffalo hump, and my bloated stomach by eating less. I just wanted to disappear, and not eating figured into that.

Since I was at a teaching hospital, every doctor's appointment became a "case" for student doctors to study me like an anatomy chart. One time I was in the hospital for extreme abdominal pains and two interns began prepping me for a gynecological exam. Upon hearing of their plans, my mom flipped out and stopped the procedure immediately. My body was no longer my own. Other people were deciding its fate. I don't know how it began, but I started to separate myself from my body; as if I were two entities in different petri dishes.

# A New Life

The treatment to save my kidneys was no longer working and my mother was told by the doctors that my situation was grave. As a result, she decided to get a second opinion. This new doctor said he would take me off all medications and put me on the waiting list for a kidney transplant. My mom got tested immediately and, by some miracle, she was a perfect match and was able to give me one of her kidneys to replace mine within a month! I had my transplant seventeen years and one day after my mom gave birth to me. I couldn't help but note the significance. With a new kidney, the Lupus went into remission. My double chin disappeared. I was thin again. Both brought equal relief.

With this new physical reality and the subsequent relief, came a sense of rebirth. And I know it sounds cheesy, but I was grateful for every breath I took. I saw life and possibility around every corner. My bookshelf began to fill with the writings of Eastern philosophers and existentialists. And I returned to yoga. It was no longer a thing my mother did. I began to practice regularly and loved it. I loved the way it made me feel physically. There were no mirrors in yoga class, so my ballet mind wasn't able to see what my body looked like. It could just be in the pose without being self-conscious. I eventually began teaching through my university. I brought humor, gratitude, and fun to my classes. I had finally found myself.

Soon my old friend perfectionism began to visit me daily. My life required it to. I had to take dozens of pills to prevent my body from rejecting my new kidney: at the same time, every day, and without fail. It was novel to be a yoga teacher at that time, and I could tell how my friends admired me. I was in a great place compared to when I was sick, but there was still this shadow that followed me. A dark side that couldn't get to a place where I could even look at, let alone accept, my inner or outer flaws. Behind it all was the fear that the Lupus would come back or my body would reject the kidney. Somehow if I wasn't perfect, my illness would return to teach me a lesson.

It took significant time to not treat my yoga practice as another form of ballet, with my head raised proud, my toes pointed, and my technique perfect. While I could do the poses just right, I wasn't fully *practicing* yoga. While others in class breathed loudly and even sighed deeply, I couldn't. I still had to keep it together. I felt silly making a noise and looked strangely at people who did. When I practiced yoga in front of my mom, she would yell, "breathe!" Yoga was not something fun to do with my body like it was when I was a child. It was something to master and control, just as I did with everything else in my life at that time.

## The Long Road to Yoga

It took me more than a decade to truly understand yoga as a spiritual practice. And when I say *yoga*, that includes yoga philosophy and meditation. Luckily, I've had many teachers, including my mother, and I learned something new about myself with each and every one.

It was Monique, a former ballet dancer, who chastised me for not "breathing right." Despite her tone, I eventually learned how to "breathe." More importantly, she taught me how to connect to my breath. Once I "discovered" my breath, the healing of my body and mind truly began. I strove to be a human "being" and stopped trying to be so perfect.

It was also in watching how hard my mom was on herself throughout the years and how she changed during her years at SRF that I witnessed how much yoga guided her into a new philosophical and spiritual place. In recalling her journey, I saw so much of myself. I realized that yoga was also my teacher and that I needed to keep practicing with the eye of a beginner to really get the most out of it. When I was angry and didn't know it, my anger was amplified on the mat. When I was sad, sometimes I cried in class. I began to notice how my emotions were ruling my state of being. And I saw that I could change the state of my negative attitude with breath and movement. I began to surrender to the moods and see them as just that: moods. I was no longer ruled by the conditions of my life.

I thought of the advice to stay with a teacher, even if you don't like them, for they have something to offer you. I recalled a former teacher who taught me compassion and gratitude. She had a hard edge, and she shared every thought in a brusque manner. One morning after our yoga class, I told her how frustrated I was over the consumerization of yoga, how it had become nothing more than a glorified exercise class. With a stern look, she said, "It doesn't matter how people get to yoga. As long as yoga is in their life they are on the path." I could feel my cheeks flush at being called out for being judgmental. She had a point. I soon realized what she said was a call for compassion and that moved me. I understood that under her hard veneer was someone who was truly on "the path," and I dropped my judgment of her, along with that of fellow yogis. I saw that there were so many different areas in my life I could bring forgiveness. I soon let compassion into my life and began a long journey of healing.

Where once my inner monologue said "You're not good enough" or "What's wrong with you?" a new voice appeared. One that answered, "It's okay, you'll be alright. No one is perfect." My mom had a long history of dealing with my perfectionism, and I realized the new voice in my head was actually hers. And a hopeful attitude washed over me.

## Forgiveness and Surrender

Where I once would do the splits and hold poses in the acrobatic forms you see on the cover of yoga magazines, I now began to stop pushing myself. I found respect for my body as this amazing home and teacher. As a result, I stopped reinjuring an ongoing problem in my back. Today, I listen to my body and judge it so much less.

With forgiveness of myself came forgiveness of and gratitude for my mother, who I had always hoped to be the perfect parent. When I was thirty-seven, she was diagnosed with stage 4 ovarian cancer. Toward the end of a long struggle with the disease, she was completely bedridden and her muscles grew incredibly tense and painful. I began doing slow movement and yoga with her. Sometimes it was just moving her arms up and down slowly with her breath. Other times I guided her through a meditation of one of her favorite memories. And other times I'd prop her up with pillows so she could be in a restorative pose. Bringing yoga to her in this way brought her great relief. And it brought me great relief. I was able to be of complete service to her and truly be present with her in a way I had longed for my whole life. We grew very close. There were no resentments and nothing left unsaid when she died. I'm so grateful to yoga for giving me this opportunity.

Today yoga is my touchstone. It is a slow and steady practice, no more fast yoga flow classes here. I don't have to do perfect acrobatic poses nor compete with myself or anyone else, for that matter. I'm much more present to the love in my life. And I am genuinely grateful for my body. At forty-four, I can do so much more with my body than I ever thought was possible. Where I once resented all that it couldn't do, I now relish what it is I am *able* to do. I am incredibly in tune with my body and listen to it every day. Some days are harder than others because I still struggle with fibromyalgia, but on the harder days I surrender. Sometimes all I can do is breathe or meditate. I trust my inner voice on a different level, and with forgiveness of myself has come an increased sense of peace.

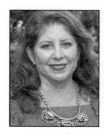

Pia Guerrero is a writer, public speaker, and leadership coach. From Harlem to Hawaii, she has led dozens of workshops and presentations on body politics, identity, intersectional feminism, media literacy, and social justice. Her work at Adios Barbie is informed by Pia's own life straddling different worlds as a bicultural Mexican and American who has never quite fit in but has finally found her home. Committed to love and justice, Pia is a yoga student/teacher and unprofessional dog walker.

Author photo by Lawrence H. Leach.

# A RECOVERED PERFECTIONIST

## *Robyn Baker*

"We don't like to tell her too many things like that. We don't want her to get a big head."

These were the words of my parents in a dimly lit therapist's office at the start of round one of inpatient treatment for anorexia at age seventeen. Growing up, my parents very rarely said anything positive about me; my schoolwork, my appearance, my talent for singing were very rarely mentioned in the form of praise or pride.

"She just always does a good job. If we start praising her, she might become full of herself."

As I sat there in a sweatshirt three sizes too big, a ghost of a girl, scared, freezing, and hopeless, all I desperately wanted to hear was how proud my parents were of me. It wasn't until years into my recovery that I would learn how the "I love yous" and the "We're so proud of yous" were only freely given when I was incredibly sick or in distress. And it wasn't until I discovered and embodied yoga that I learned how that price point was more than I was ever willing to pay again.

# The Roots of Perfectionism

I grew up living a very privileged life; both of my parents worked in education and made a good living, and we never had to go without, or at least I never noticed if we did. I also grew up with thin privilege; I never experienced being bullied or teased for my appearance or lack of ability. I was never considered overweight and, as a child, was never concerned about my size. Teachers and mentors would constantly praise my accomplishments, talents, and my "exotic" appearance. Being a mixed race child in the 1980s was pretty rare (and not as accepted as it is today). I was an outgoing child and loved singing and musical theater.

I was the exact opposite of my older brother, who struggled in school, had few friends, was very much introverted, and didn't participate in many after-school activities. My brother was frequently in trouble with my father for one thing or another, and witnessing the yelling, violence, and punishments he would receive led my young mind to a simple and nearly deadly conclusion: Be perfect and your parents will love you.

I have read that perfectionism is deeply rooted in the DNA of certain unfortunate souls, but I would argue that sometimes it can also be environmental and a learned trait; I believe I was a result of both. The perfectionism I applied to my talents and abilities as a child out of fear of getting punished eventually found its way to my body when I reached high school. During my senior year, life was out of control; I was traveling across the country to audition for performing arts colleges, my sleep was nonexistent between the loads of homework and the hours of rehearsals for the various shows I was participating in, and, above all of this, I still didn't feel perfect enough to receive the love of my parents. My father's alcoholism made my home life unpredictable and scary to say the least.

My body was the one thing I could control in a world that felt impossible to deal with. Under the influence of the endless weight-loss marketing campaigns promising me happiness at the end of a ten-pound weight loss rainbow coupled with the anxiety and depression brought on by the internal and external pressure to live up to expectations as a straight A student, talented performer, and perfectly sized teenager, I decided it was time to go on a diet. You know, just to feel better about myself, and maybe everything in my world would get better once I lost a few pounds because that's what I was being promised; look "better" and your life will be better.

As I began to shrink in size from a lack of adequate nutrition and hydration, I felt strangely empowered and strong. The constant dull ache of hunger helped to numb the other negative feelings in my life and it was an intoxicating sense of relief. When well-intended compliments on my increasingly smaller body from classmates and teachers filled the gaping hole that made up my lack of self-worth and self-esteem, I became addicted. The game of how low could I make the number on the scale go became the one and only thing that mattered and made me feel at peace. Six months later, I was in the hospital nearly dead from anorexia.

## The Cost of Chasing the Perfect Body

My first round of in-patient treatment for my eating disorder was a joke. Not only was the program inadequate, I was anything but open and/or committed to receiving the help I was being offered. I was discharged early in order to graduate high school, and I had little to no skills as to how to reenter a "normal" teenage life. I was still fervently counting each calorie that passed my lips, scared to death of weight gain, far below a healthy weight zone, and suffering from a terrible body image. The outlook was not great.

My drive to "perfect" my physical appearance was still the engine fueling my destructive actions. With eating disorders being as tricky and manipulating as they come, I soon found a way to disguise my need for body perfection as a step forward in my recovery. I took up weight lifting. With weight gain ordered by my treatment team, weight lifting seemed like the perfect solution to not only help me gain weight through building muscle, but it also gave me yet another way I could control my body and not be fat (which is what my eating disorder feared more than death). I would sculpt the perfect body from the ground up and everyone would think I was being healthy because my so-called objective would be to add muscle.

My eating disorder and I were in heaven.

I developed a strict and lengthy weight-lifting regimen, which eventually spiraled off into indoor cycling classes and hours spent on the elliptical trainer, obsessively gripping an illusion of something that would make living tolerable and give my existence meaning: the "perfect" body. Yes, there were the rare moments where an honest desire to get off this endless hamster wheel of self-destruction existed. But along with each hopeful thought, ten well-intended but harmful compliments about my dedication, discipline, and "perfect body" would instantly change my mind. It was like making a decision to climb a mountain only to be directed back down after two steps because of bad weather. Eventually, the gym where I fulfilled my obsession hired me as a personal trainer. The manager suggested I work there since I was there so much already, after all. I was hired without an interview or any formal training—just an unrelenting and fanatical obsession with exercise and a steadfast belief that my body would be worthless and unacceptable without it (which in turn would make me a failure and unlovable).

I believed I had finally obtained the perfect socially acceptable system for controlling my body and mind to ultimately obtain a sense of self-worth and importance. The compliments I continued to receive on a daily basis strengthened my disordered thinking and behaviors. Underneath this false sense of superiority and confidence, I *desperately wanted out.* But I knew what it would cost me to leave; it meant abandoning all I had worked for, including my level of success as a personal trainer and Pilates instructor, a feeling of absolute certainty that my life would be intolerable, and that I would lose everything that gave me a sense of not only control but also importance and meaning. My so-called "perfect" body was everything to me and losing it would be more than I thought I could humanly tolerate.

What I didn't realize was that underneath it all my body was literally collapsing in on itself. I developed a stress fracture in my hip as a result of the endless pounding of pavement from the hours of running I forced myself to do in order to gain permission to eat. After a bone density scan, I was told that at the age of twenty-four I had developed osteoporosis and my bones were that of a seventy-year-old. Regardless, my obsession continued as I spiraled further downward... until an intervention was orchestrated by my parents and therapist. As a result, I entered back into treatment ten years after the onset of my eating disorder.

## There Is No Perfect Pose

Entering treatment for a second time, I knew what to expect, and I also knew that it was up to me to decide whether or not I was going to work the program and commit to recovery. No one else could do it but me. I was sick and tired of being sick and tired; I had lost my dream of performing, my high school sweetheart, and, most importantly, my health. The fear of losing more of my life finally became greater than the fear of losing control over my socially defined "perfect" body. The unknown outcome of committing to recovery finally became the lesser of two evils.

Initially, all forms of exercise were banned during inpatient treatment, as weight stabilization and weight gain were my prescribed objective. But as my health improved and my mental outlook shifted, I was slowly reintroduced to exercise. I was able to do weight lifting, Nia (a form of dance exercise), and, of course, yoga. Of all three exercise options, yoga was my least favorite. I had practiced yoga a few times at the gym where I worked, but I was not a fan. In fact, the only reason I walked into a yoga class in the first place was because my therapist had suggested that I do it on my "rest day" in order to feel like I was still doing something.

I truly couldn't stand yoga; it was slow, it was relaxing (which was not what I wanted at the time), and it made my blood boil over with anxiety because I thought I could burn more calories elsewhere than during a single yoga session. Yes, I was committed to my recovery, but the thought of focusing on my breath instead of pushing myself to fatigue or perform the best out of everyone in the class was so incredibly foreign and frustrating to me that I wanted to scream.

The words of the instructor irked me more than anything. Preaching things like, "allow your body to release into the pose" or "there is no perfect pose, so explore what feels best to you" only made me roll my eyes with annoyance.

*Of course there is a perfect pose! I can do the pose with prefect form, I am the most flexible and I will be the best at this yoga thing*, were all silent responses to my teacher's little nuggets of wisdom. The worst was when the teacher asked us to be present in our body; doing any such thing was not only something that sounded completely uncomfortable to me, but I didn't have the slightest idea as to how to actually do it. Plus, with my needed weight gain and feeling my clothes gripping tighter onto my newly expanding body, all I desperately wanted to do was escape my body. The truth was I hadn't been present in my body for more than a decade, and I didn't have the slightest idea as to what that even meant. Starvation and my obsessive exercise habits had served to numb the connection between my body and my self. Healing this connection was going to take a lot of time as well as a willingness, which didn't come until years after I was discharged.

## Breathing into Imperfection

Against my treatment team's recommendations, I eventually made my way back to the fitness industry about a year after being discharged from treatment. They likened my decision as similar to that of the alcoholic working in a bar. I knew it was a risky move, but it was the only thing I could see myself doing for work.

I once again began working as a certified Pilates instructor at a high-end gym and was able to remain in recovery, but it wasn't easy. With self-imposed body shaming comments coming from clients, mirrors reflecting my image everywhere I turned, and the temptation to fall into the body comparison game, I knew I would have to work incredibly hard to maintain my recovery.

Although my relationship with exercise was still one that I would classify as "it's complicated," I was able to stay within the activity parameters set out for me by my team of doctors and therapists. The compulsive urge to literally kill myself through my workouts had dissipated. In its place was a sense of caution and apprehension toward exercise. I did not trust myself nor could I properly identify when I had physically done "enough" without relying on a time limit or the number of sets and repetitions completed. The connection between my body and my self was still nonexistent. Without a quest for the "perfect body" or the need to numb out, my exercise felt aimless and boring. And without the ability to intuitively listen to and be present within my body, my recovery was not yet complete. This is when I happened to rediscover yoga.

I was persuaded to try out yoga by a fellow instructor I had befriended at the gym. She hit the right button when she said I would be great at yoga since I was such a master at Pilates. Under that influence of my ego telling me I would be better than the other students, I decided to give yoga another shot. I had no expectations going in and told myself I would do it just this one time to satisfy the wishes of my friend (and my ego). At one point during the class, we held warrior two for what seemed like forever. As my legs began to shake, I attempted to distract my mind away from the fatigue by thinking of my day ahead and other "monkey mind" thoughts. Just then the instructor called out something that changed my life forever, "Get comfortable with feeling uncomfortable." Was she actually asking to me to pay attention to my fatigue and be okay with it? If I were to do that, how would I ever make it through the class? Disconnecting between my body and my self was what I did, and I was damn good at it.

For purely perfectionistic and ego-satisfying reasons, I went back for more yoga classes. Eventually, I decided to follow the instructor's cue by attempting to focus on taking deeper breaths in order to stay present in my body. All my mind wanted to do was escape the sensation of fatigue, but as I deepened my breath and felt a sense of calm circulating through my body, I discovered for the first time how to practice allowing my body to physically feel uncomfortable and accept it.

The experience felt real and authentic ... and it felt like coming *home*.

This experience felt different from the rules established by my treatment team and the lists of coping skills I was told to use if I wanted to remain in my recovery. It was as if my body was telling me everything was going to be okay and that I could trust this process. I didn't have to tune out the discomfort and remain numb. I could sit with it, breathe, and come to center (and even feel calm). It didn't happen overnight, in fact it didn't happen within a year, but I eventually discovered that if I could mentally stay present and calm within physical discomfort (be it holding warrior two for eternity or feeling "gross" in my body), I could do the same with my uncomfortable thoughts and feelings. And with practice, just like with the physical practice of yoga, over time the thoughts and feelings that once caused me emotional and mental discomfort became easier to tolerate and let go of.

## Creating Perfectly Authentic Work

Eleven years after I was first inducted into the trigger-filled fitness industry via obsession and self-destruction, I came to realize I could no longer pretend that what I was doing was okay. Performing "fitness evolutions" on new members, which included taking their circumference measurements, testing their body fat, and, of course, weighing them on the scale, was completely against everything I had come to believe in and physically stand for. I tolerated it for a painstaking amount of time until one day I was pushed over the edge by a comment I couldn't ignore.

I was working with a client who was compulsively exercising and asking me to assist her to drop body fat to unhealthy levels. After refusing several times to help her with this, I spoke with her physician, who encouraged me to help her with her body fat goals even after admitting she probably needed help but that there were worse things she could be addicted to. I remembered my yoga and breathed when all I wanted to do was scream at him and cry. It was time for me to create my own space where I could not only guide others through exercise in a body-positive and self-empowering atmosphere but also preserve my own sanity and, most of all, my recovery. The fear of leaving a steady job and going out on my own was on par with going back into treatment, but I knew in my heart it was what I had to do. I knew it was going to be scary, unpredictable, and difficult, and if it wasn't for the wisdom and trust I gained through my yoga practice, I would have never had the courage to trust my inner wisdom that everything was going to be okay. No matter what the outcome, trusting and honoring my true self, which I had cultivated and connected to through yoga, was always the right answer.

## There Is No Perfection, Just Happiness

Our bodies and our lives are in constant flux. As I sit here today, a business owner of the only body-positive and recovery-centered fitness studio in Orange County, California, my belly round and full at the halfway point of my second pregnancy, I must admit that change, especially physical change, can still be a difficult beast. Many times, I feel like I've finally made complete peace with my body, only to realize I haven't because out of the blue maybe a dress doesn't fit quite the same way or I discover a patch of stretch marks on the back of my legs that I didn't know existed or a well-intended client makes some slight remark about the size of my body and the negative thoughts and emotions attempt to squeeze their way back into the forefront of my mind. It is then that my yoga reminds me not only to breathe and get comfortable with feeling uncomfortable, but also that the things I see and hear about my body are not real nor are they definitive markers of the quality of my heart or the essence of my spirit. And, with that, I am reminded that maintaining a positive and peaceful relationship with my body is an ongoing practice. It's not an end point or final destination.

There is no such thing as a "perfect pose" and there is no such thing as the "perfect body" that will bestow endless happiness. The "perfect body" and, really, the "perfect life" is what you choose at that moment. The most beautiful thing about that is you can *decide* it is you right now in this very moment! And that happiness and peace can be obtained without any social media likes or words of praise from parents or others. Choosing happiness is choosing to decide everything in your life, including your body, is perfect in this moment *and every moment*.

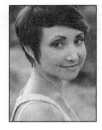

Robyn Baker is the owner and operator of Asteya Fitness, Orange County's only body-positive fitness studio. After recovering from a decade-long battle with anorexia and exercise addiction, during which she worked as a personal trainer and Pilates instructor, Robyn decided to return to the fitness industry in hopes of changing the way people think about and approach exercise by challenging and someday ending the insidious body-shaming messages propagated within the fitness community. She holds a BS in Kinesiology and is certified in Yoga, Pilates, and Personal Training.

Author photo by Austin O'Brien Photography.

# SAYING GOOD-BYE
# TO THE INNER CRITIC

*Dr. Melissa Mercedes*

There is something daunting about not feeling comfortable in your own body and skin. Whether this discomfort stems from a disruption in the attachment process as an infant or dissatisfaction with body weight, shape, or size due to mass consumption of media portrayals of what constitutes the "perfect body" is important. Equally or perhaps even more important, though, is how we choose to respond to the situation.

Body image is defined as one's cognitive, emotional, and behavioral reactions to body weight and shape.[1] Research suggests that body image dissatisfaction is learned not only through the media's portrayal of what is acceptable, but also through familial factors (e.g., teasing by family members, family's emphasis on weight) and social comparisons. Social contextual factors such as Western culture's emphasis on the ultra-thin body and peer influence informs the construction of an unrealistic ideal of what is beautiful. Our cultural ideal of thinness seems to be, in part, predicated on the waif-thin appearance popularized in the 1990s.

1. Tiggeman and Lynch, "Body Appreciation in Adult Women: Relationships with Age and Body Satisfaction," *Elsevier*, 2001. https://www.6minutes.com.au /getmedia/78426d7b-f84e-46af-bb17-de4e6c51d6a9/body-image-paper.aspx.

Since the 1960s, the ideal female shape has become smaller and thinner. Hence, Western society is bombarded by a body image ideal that is, in large part, overly unrealistic and nearly impossible to attain. The influence of media, coupled with family and peer influences, is the backdrop for the stories we continuously tell ourselves, often subconsciously, about our body shape and weight in the context of what is attractive. Unfortunately, these stories have no age boundaries and can traverse a lifetime, well into our forties, fifties, and beyond.

As a teenager in high school, I was introduced to the modeling industry. Here, I was exposed to a different perspective on food and body image. I learned how to design low-calorie meals and successfully skip meals. I was convinced that I needed to lose ten to fifteen pounds, because the camera apparently adds this much weight to your body in photographs. That message ran deep. It was during this time that I began to cultivate and nurture perfectionistic tendencies linked to a persistent delusion of an ideal body put forth by the media and based on social comparisons. I became captivated by the media's portrayal of the "healthy" female body, and I blindly followed a path marked by an unhealthy relationship to food and body. I became addicted to a story: I am not skinny enough, and until I achieve a certain weight and body mass index, I will not be worthy. Eventually my life became extremely narrow as I obsessed over calories and the types of food I ate.

I became stuck on the notion that I had to make drastic changes to my body if I was going to be successful in the industry. What I did not understand at the time was that I was fighting an uphill battle if this was the intended outcome. Why? Because it was not that I was "overweight," but rather, I had a body shape and size that was different from the media's ideal. I am of Mexican, German, and Aztec decent—I do not inhabit the tall, slender body frame that was sought by the modeling industry. Being an unenlightened consumer of the mass media and trained to compare myself to peers, I became stuck. To be successful in the industry, I would have to step into a completely different body.

Over time, I began to develop deep-rooted thoughts that I was unacceptable or unworthy in some way. To appease these thoughts, I engaged in unhealthy eating behaviors. The ramifications of this new perspective was reflected in my dis-ease in the body. I spent my teenage years and early twenties learning how to avoid the experience of fully inhabiting my body, missing the opportunity to dwell in the place where we go to connect to our inner guidance, strength, and self-love. I became habituated to avoiding the discomfort associated with a delusional body image, and I resisted any opportunity to experience what it felt like to be in my own skin. Not surprising, no matter how much weight I lost, the shape and height of my body remained the same. More importantly, the weight loss failed to bring me the happiness, self-love, and acceptance that, according to the billboards, magazines, and television commercials, comes with drastic weight loss and attaining the ideal weight.

While the seeds of dissatisfaction with body image were planted during my teenage years, it was in my twenties when those seeds manifested into a personal medical condition that could not be ignored. This was the wake-up call that ignited the fire within to start looking at my unhealthy relationship with food and body and the desire to find that one diet or trick that would "fix" my body. I relied primarily on Eastern traditions to support my healing process, which marks the beginning of a spiritual journey that continues to offer support, nurturance, and guidance both personally and professionally.

## Waking Up to Presence

I took my first yoga class at a gym in 1999. What I remember from that experience was this overwhelming feeling of being safe in my body for the first time ever. It felt as though I had come back home and stepped into this beautiful sanctuary that was my body, and I never wanted to leave. This left a significant imprint on my mind, and I was inspired to delve deeper into the asana practice as well as into the philosophy of this ancient practice. I became so enticed by the beauty of the practice and its healing effects that I eventually signed up for a nine-week yoga teacher training. It was during this time that I also began to explore Vipassana meditation at Spirit Rock Meditation Center in Woodacre, California.

I saw the meditation practice as a great complement to my yoga practice. These Eastern traditions provided the opportunity to learn how to watch thoughts, without becoming entangled or attached, and to create space from the thoughts as you gently guide your way back to the present moment without judgment, evaluation, or criticism. The movement associated with breath in the yoga asana practice provided a unique platform upon which to cultivate and strengthen mindfulness skills. Through the asana practice, I began to notice that there is always a choice point of staying on my mat despite the experience of uncomfortable mental phenomenon and to draw on the breath as a focal point. Or to drown in the mental chatter and become lost in the story associated with the thoughts and emotions. The asana practice also allowed me to engage in exposure rather than avoidance. When I stepped onto my mat, found my breath, and moved through the asanas, I developed willingness to remain in contact with the internal experiences centered on body-related thoughts, feelings, and emotions. Such experiences that were initially perceived to be scary and uncomfortable and led to resistance. Through the exposure, I learned that if I did not give energy to what my mind was feeding me, it would eventually subside. For so many years, I identified with these dysfunctional body image–related thoughts and ideas, and somehow I convinced myself that it was truth. This faulty belief system I created for myself and operated within had led to misguided and misdirected behaviors.

Mindfulness skills such as noticing, accepting, and surrendering enabled me to recognize hunger cues, to "sit with" the feeling of satiety, and to allow the associated physiological responses to arise without resistance or interference that often took the form of compensatory behaviors. Further, the consistent intentional practice of greeting the present moment with a stance of openness and acceptance was fundamental to my healing process.

My meditation practice during this time focused on loving-kindness and compassion. Traditionally, loving-kindness meditation is practiced toward self, first, and is then directed toward other people in your life. The main tenet of this practice is to cultivate a sense of connection with all people through principles of generosity and nonharming. The most difficult aspect of this practice for me was offering loving-kindness toward myself. Notably, though, this was also the most rewarding in addressing the distorted beliefs about my body and to reach a place of unconditional love and acceptance.

The practice of compassion also helped me to understand the many ways in which I became stuck in the negative psychological states of fear and anxiety surrounding my body. Rather than approach with curiosity and openness, I chose to avoid and turn away from these present moment experiences. The integration of compassion with my practice allowed me to cultivate forgiveness and patience, which, in turn, engendered a stance of openness and acceptance to whatever was unfolding from moment to moment. Over time, I was able to distance myself from the thought that there was something inherently wrong with me and, more importantly, that I had somehow "given up" when I stopped letting negative thought patterns dictate my behaviors.

The exposure to discomfort and staying with the discomfort, embedded in both meditation and yoga, offered a pathway to healthy and organic change from within. I came into this place of acceptance and opening to the phenomenon that thoughts will arise, fall, and arise again, and I was no longer controlled by the ebb and flow of thought, emotion, and sensation surrounding body image. When we consistently open ourselves to an unpleasant situation, whether it is in the form of a negative thought about our body or physical sensation, over time we learn that nonresistance to what is unfolding in that moment can bring freedom from attachment to the story embedded in our minds. These insights were followed by the epiphany: "If this beautiful process is unfolding on my yoga mat and meditation pillow, how can it be translated into our everyday life situations?"

## Holding the Light for Others

My personal and spiritual experiences coalesced into a path of self-discovery filled with endless possibilities, not only to do work on the inside, but also to step into that place where I can be of highest service to others. The possibility to integrate personal and spiritual experiences with science to inform and effect change through research and clinical work on women's health issues was the impetus to pursue a PhD in clinical psychology. I am now a licensed clinical psychologist, and my research and clinical work is focused on women's mental health and mind-body therapies for depression, anxiety, body image issues, and trauma.

I was afraid to remain in contact with private internal experiences that took the form of disturbing thoughts, emotions, and physical sensations pertaining to my body shape and size. Stepping onto my mat day after day and staying with the discomfort provided insight into the function of these behavioral tendencies (i.e., emotional avoidance and the role of yoga and meditation as conduits to psychological healing). The motivation to further explore these relationships in my work with women was cultivated to some degree by what transpired through the Eastern practices. Loving-kindness and compassion practices not only brought awareness to the subtle ways in which I was being dictated by society's construction of how a woman should look in her body, but also the powerful shifts that can emerge through the simple act of becoming still, both mentally and physically. Attempts to fit the media's portrayal of the perfect body type or to try and fight against the natural flow of thoughts and emotions were fruitless. The transformational change I witnessed fueled my desire to integrate these teachings with Western psychology, with an aim to provide others with tools for turning internal chaos into something meaningful in their lives.

Before enrolling in graduate school, I taught yoga full time and was involved with research on women and depression. I recall having conversations with female yoga students about various women's health-related issues, ranging from mood and anxiety during pregnancy and postpartum to dysfunctional relationships with body and food. An underlying theme of the latter seemed to be a lack of self-acceptance and a constant striving to look a different way. Within the scientific community, theoretical models of disordered eating and body image dissatisfaction conceptualize the function of unhealthy eating behaviors or emphasis on body image as ways to achieve emotional avoidance. Notably, body image dissatisfaction is a national epidemic with prevalence rates ranging from 11 percent to 72 percent[2] and is a key determinant of eating disorders.

The desire to support women in addressing body image issues dovetailed into a passion to explore the integration of yoga and meditation with Western psychology. For my dissertation, I developed a yoga program for women with postpartum depression, which helped to improve women's symptoms of depression and anxiety, along with their overall quality of life.

Subsequent clinical and research endeavors provided the opportunity to further hone my work in women veteran's mental health, and to focus on the development and implementation of yoga and mindfulness programs for women veterans. There is a growing body of research documenting the benefits of mindfulness and yoga for negative psychological states such as anxiety, depression, and stress, as well as for medical conditions, including chronic pain. Further, newer forms of psychotherapies are being developed that pull from Eastern philosophies, such as Buddhism, and focus on integrating the key tenets of mindfulness. These newer therapies, referred to as "third-wave" therapies, are arguably successful in their ability to help individuals become less attached to their struggles and ultimately move into life situations with more joy and vitality and less suffering. The integration of mindfulness and meditation with Western psychology helps to broaden a person's behavioral repertoire to consider the context in which the behavior is occurring and provides an opportunity for the person to better understand the function of other behaviors outside of the present situation.

The integration of my personal and professional experiences has allowed me to cultivate awareness and the power within to transform my relationship to food and body. My spiritual practice shed light on the many ways in which I became entangled with the misconceptions of what my body should look like, primarily dictated by societal norms. My work as a clinical psychologist helped to further develop my insight

2. Fiske, et al., "Prevalence of Body Dissatisfaction Among United States Adults" *Eating Behaviors* 15(3), 2014. https://www.researchgate.net/publication/262304198 _Prevalence_of_Body_Dissatisfaction_Among_United_States_Adults_Review_and _Recommendations_for_Future_Research.

into the connections between the identification with negative thoughts about body size and shape, and maladaptive behaviors that served to perpetuate my dysfunctional relationship with self. Through these pathways, I learned how to embrace my divine uniqueness regardless of body shape, size, and weight. My personal journey continues to fuel the passion for my work in a beautiful and magical way. From this place, I am now able to help guide others toward meaningful lives filled with love and acceptance and less suffering. For this, I am deeply grateful.

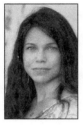

Melissa Mercedes, PhD, is a licensed clinical psychologist and conducts clinical research at the VA Greater Los Angeles and San Diego Healthcare Systems. She has extensive experience in the use of mind-body therapies for trauma, depression, and anxiety in women, and is an advocate for integrative approaches to promote emotional and physical well-being.

Author photo by Naru Photography.

# KRIYA YOGA—LIVING YOGA

## Jivana Heyman

We all have transformational moments in our lives. Those single moments that you can picture so clearly when so many other moments are a blur. I remember one moment when I was about twelve or thirteen, standing in the hall of the house I grew up in, and realizing that I wasn't like the rest of my family—I was gay.

Thankfully, these days it doesn't seem like such a big deal to be gay. But, in the late seventies it still was. I didn't have any positive role models for what it meant to be a gay man—other than Charles Nelson Reilly on Match Game. In that moment, standing in the hall, I remember a feeling of great sadness, grief actually, over the mistaken belief that I wouldn't be able to have a family and that I wouldn't have children. I felt sure that I would spend my life alone and isolated from all the things that seemed to offer comfort and security. I had no idea that those things would be possible for me.

I hated my body for being attracted to men. I felt that it had betrayed me, and it was leading me to a sad and lonely life. Ironically, gay men are stereotyped as narcissistic, yet my experience was the exact opposite. How could I love my body, which was the source of so much confusion, pain, and sadness? My body was drawing me away from everything that society was telling me that I needed to be happy—a loving partner and a family.

I came out when I was seventeen, and so did my self-hatred. I was finally being honest about who I was, but it didn't translate into self-acceptance. Instead, my first relationships with other men were desperate attempts for validation. I couldn't see myself. It was like I was a ghost, and I would haunt any man who was attracted to me. I would sleep with anyone who showed any interest in me at all, because I was desperate for some kind of acceptance—anything that looked like love. Eventually, I dated one man in college for more than a year, but he finally left me because he said I was just too needy.

On top of my own self-hatred, society was turning against gay men as the fear of AIDS exploded in the late eighties. Suddenly, dear friends and lovers were getting sick and dying. I was living in San Francisco and working with ACT UP, the AIDS activist group, as well as volunteering at a local AIDS hospice. It was an incredibly sad and painful time; I was in my early twenties—finally out of the closet—and surrounded by illness and death. This reality shifted my thinking from the normal twenty-something's musings to deep questions about life, death, and spirituality.

Luckily, I had recently rediscovered yoga and stumbled into a yoga class with an Integral Yoga teacher in Berkeley. I say "rediscovered" because my grandmother had a strong daily yoga practice—she was way ahead of her time. When I was young, I would watch her practicing in the mornings and sometimes join in. I remember looking at poses in her yoga book with a man with a gold face on the cover. When I rediscovered yoga in my early twenties, my teacher had this same book, and I realized that my grandmother had also studied Integral Yoga with Swami Satchidananda—the book was *Integral Yoga Hatha*, his classic yoga textbook.

Yoga crept up on me. I was busy with my activism, but I found myself drawn more and more to meditation and the subtle practices of yoga, which offered a new experience of deep connection. Through yoga, my self-image began to shift. I remember one day my yoga teacher stopped me after class and said, "You know, you don't have to live like this." For a long time, I had no idea what she meant. I was so used to being angry—hating my body for being attracted to men, hating the world for its homophobia, and for killing my friends with AIDS. I didn't know how else to live.

As I began to practice more, I could feel my body changing. After years of severe digestive problems, I could feel the knot in my belly loosening. But it wasn't all positive. One day in an advanced asana class, I pulled too hard in a forward bend and *boom* I could barely move. I had torn my SI joint, and I would spend years healing it. My self-hatred had found its way into my practice as I pushed beyond my limits. Healing was slow, but I knew that in yoga I had found a balm to sooth my pain.

The pain of my youth was a form of *tapas*—purification through suffering. In the *Yoga Sutras*, the great sage Patanjali says the first step in practicing yoga is accepting the suffering in our lives as a catalyst for growth. Rather than feel victimized by what life throws at us, we say okay to the challenges of life and use the suffering as fuel for self-awareness. It is those challenging moments, and the way we respond to them, that help to shape the form of our lives and even create our destiny. This is what was happening to me—slowly I was beginning to accept the suffering rather than fight it, and the result was brief moments of peace unlike any I had known.

In Book 2, Sutra 1, of the *Yoga Sutras*, Patanjali follows *tapas* with two more teachings: *svadhyaya* (reflection) and *ishvara pranidhana* (faith). This yoga trifecta has magical powers of transformation, as we learn to move from pain to peace.

## *Svadhyaya:* Reflection

I soon found myself training at the San Francisco Integral Yoga Institute to become a yoga teacher, and I was mesmerized by the yoga teachings. The concept of *svadhyaya* was new to me—the idea of witnessing my mind rather than being the thoughts. This meant that I could begin to look honestly and openly at the way my mind was working. What a gift. Previously, I felt victimized by my own relentless negative and critical thoughts. Then, I started to realize that I could step back and observe the thoughts instead of *being* them.

In 1995, I started sharing yoga with the HIV/AIDS community in San Francisco, and I taught in local hospitals. I was struck by my students' reactions to the yoga teachings. So many of them seemed to be on a spiritual fast track, speeding through life lessons that normally take decades to learn. It was an incredible gift to spend time learning from them as they faced the reality of death—some in utter fear and some in peace. I wondered what allowed some people to die so peacefully. How could they come to such a deep acceptance when death is so terrifying?

According to Swami Satchidananda, our true nature is happiness, and any unhappiness or stress we experience is caused by our attachments—things outside of ourselves that we think we need to be happy. An attachment can be shallow or deep: shallow like wanting to buy a new shirt or deep like the desperate need for someone to love us. The ties that bind us are created in our mind. We tether ourselves to these things in a desperate attempt to be happy when, in fact, it's the tethering, the desiring, that is keeping us down. It's the desires themselves that cause the unhappiness.

Non-attachment, on the other hand, is freedom from these endless desires: the experience of universal love. As the *Bhagavad Gita* explains, it is freedom from "the wishing and selfishness fever." [1] This concept of non-attachment became a touchstone in my life when my closest friend, Kurt, died of AIDS in 1995. Kurt was a student of yoga philosophy, and he loved the concept of non-attachment. He said that it encapsulated all the spiritual teachings in one simple idea—releasing the material world and holding on to Love.

A few months before his death, Kurt knew that his time on earth was limited, and he decided to approach death with a sense of inquiry and reflection that is the core of *svadhyaya*. He was a writer and lover of lists. When we would spend time together, he would inevitably start making a list about something, "Let's think of all the places you've ever lived," or "Name all of the people you've dated." So I wasn't surprised when Kurt announced that as a way to wrestle with death, he was going

---

1. Easwaran Eknath, *The Bhagavad Gita* (Petaluma, CA: Nilgiri Press, 1985).

to make a daily list of all his attachments—things he needed from the world to be happy.

At first, his list of attachments was very long. After a few days, he announced that he got his list down to just four things:

1. His partner

2. His dog

3. His apartment (he did live in San Francisco after all)

4. Me, his best friend (I was honored to make the top four!)

For a few weeks, he was stuck on those four, and he couldn't seem to get the list any shorter. Then he got really sick: He had Kaposi sarcoma, skin lesions, all over his body and face. He had lymphoma, which made his face so swollen that he was unrecognizable, and he had retinitis, which made him blind. He was in the hospital for weeks, and one day when I went to visit him, I was surprised to see that he was in a very good mood. He said that he was happy because he got his list of attachments down to just two things:

1. His partner

2. His dog

I was a little taken aback by this announcement. I was off the list. I asked him why that was a good thing, because it kind of felt like I was being abandoned. He turned to me and said, "You are my dear spiritual friend. I love you, and we'll always be together."

I still didn't get it. I kept visiting him in the hospital as he got sicker and sicker. One day he slipped into a coma, and then he died the next day. He was never able to reduce his lists of attachments, and for good reason. Both his partner and his dog relied on him so much and both of them really suffered after his death.

Surprisingly, I had the opposite experience. I expected to be devastated when Kurt died because he was the friend who was always there for me, listening to me, and taking care of me. But, for some reason, I was okay. Kurt's love stayed with me in a way that I didn't think was possible. Kurt's conscious good-bye was deeply healing for me on a subtle level. He taught me what non-attachment really was—deep, pure, unselfish Love.

## *Ishvara Pranidhana:* Faith

Yoga was doing its magic. By 1997, I had been with my partner, Matt, for four years. Our relationship was getting stronger, and we wanted to build a family together. I found I had a new faith that I had never experienced before.

We wanted to have a commitment ceremony (the idea of gay marriage didn't even exist yet!), and we thought that the Integral Yoga Institute would be the perfect location. Of course, there had never been a gay marriage at the Institute, and no one knew what Swami Satchidananda would think of the idea. Luckily, he was visiting San Francisco about six months before the date that we were considering for the ceremony, so I had an opportunity to ask him in person.

Generally, Swami Satchidananda was a busy guy, and the only time I had the chance to speak with him was when he was at the airport, arriving or departing. In those days, you could go right up to the gate, even if you didn't have a ticket. So, in the airport I waited in a long line of people who were going up and speaking to him about all their various problems. Nervously, I asked him if it was okay for Matt and I to get married at the Institute. His response was, "Okay, when?"

I was a little surprised by his immediate positive response, and I muttered, "Well, we're thinking of August 31." Then I moved away and many other people came up to speak with him. About half an hour later, he got up to board his plane and walked over to me. He looked me in the eye and said, "August 31st, I'll be thinking of you." I was blown away by his loving acceptance and the fact that he remembered the date from our earlier discussion. In that moment, I felt that I was finally being seen after a life of invisibility.

## The Yoga of Parenting

In the following years, Matt and I adopted two children through open adoption, and now they are fifteen and eleven. I was working as a yoga teacher, and so my schedule gave me the flexibility to stay home with the kids when they were little. I feel blessed to have had the experience of being the main caregiver, which most men don't get to do. Yet, parenting was, and continues to be, the most challenging experience of my life.

It's easy for me to be peaceful when I'm alone, to do my practice, and get quiet inside. It's harder for me to keep that peace in the face of daily life. When my daughter is angry about something at school and turns that anger toward me, it takes a lot of self-awareness to remain neutral enough to see the dynamic unfolding rather than reacting. This is the secret power of yoga—helping us keep calm in the storm.

In my daughter's adolescent mind, I see a reflection of my own self-doubt and insecurity. The pressure on girls and women to be good at everything (and look amazing while doing it) is preposterous. When it gets to be too much, she goes for self-doubt and self-criticism or she lashes out. I worry about her self-image and wonder how yoga can help her to stay connected in a disconnected digital world.

The other day, she called herself fat and I didn't know how to react. On the one hand, denying it and saying, "Oh, no, you're not fat," is simply playing into her body issues. Instead, I asked her why she said that and if she feels pressure to look a certain way. She laughed it off, as she often does whenever I start getting philosophical. But the issues are impossible to avoid. She wants to buy makeup and go shopping for clothes all the time, but I notice in the midst of shopping there is a basic unhappiness there. Shopping brings up the insecurities, and even though we shield her as much as possible from the media, she is mesmerized by the media's messages around self-worth, beauty, and the roles of women and girls.

I try to balance those messages with a different story. The messages I give her come out of my own experience of healing from self-hatred. I tell her that each of us is a spark of the Divine. We each have special skills and talents that are needed in the world. Our job is to uncover that special calling and embrace ourselves, regardless of what the world is telling us.

As parents, we need yoga even more. We have such a difficult line to walk, and I think we end up sending mixed messages to our kids. We want our kids to listen to us and behave a certain way, yet we want them to be free and to be true to themselves. It's like we're saying "Be yourself ... but only the version I want you to be." What is incredible about yoga is that it gives parents the tools we need to connect with the truth within ourselves so we don't look to our children to fulfill our needs.

Ironically, the actual teaching about yoga and body image is that we're not the body. Swami Sivananda used to sing, "I'm not the body, not the mind, immortal Self I am!" Connecting with the immortal Self sounds daunting, but that's really what yoga is about. My goal is not simply to teach my kids yoga, but to teach them that there is a way to connect with the immortal Self. Once we are connected there, we can find a balanced relationship with our physical body—a balanced relationship of acceptance and gratitude.

Being a friend, parent, and partner has offered me so many lessons that sitting in meditation could only begin to teach me. The challenges of coming out as a teenager, losing my friends in my twenties, and parenting through my thirties and forties has helped me learn more about myself. I see that my challenges are opportunities for growth (*tapas*). If I reflect on what I'm learning I see where I'm attached (*svadhyaya*), and eventually I see that the answer is always to let go, have faith, and connect with love (*ishvara pranidhana*).

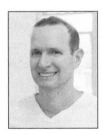

Jivana Heyman is the founder of Accessible Yoga, which is an international organization dedicated to sharing yoga with all. Currently, Accessible Yoga offers annual conferences, teacher training programs around the world, ambassador programs, and an online directory. Jivana is also co-owner of the Santa Barbara Yoga Center, manager of the San Francisco Integral Yoga Institute, and is an Integral Yoga Minister. His passion is making yoga accessible to everyone and empowering people with the yoga practices. For more information visit www.accessibleyoga.org.

Author photo by Sarit Z Rogers.

# ON LIVING BOLD AND DISCOVERING YOUR POWER

*Dr. Jenny Copeland*

I have a confession to make: I have only been practicing asana, the physical element of yoga, for about two years. But yoga as a whole? I think that has been present in my heart from the very beginning.

## Searching

With few exceptions, I spent much of my time growing up being the skinniest person in the room. I have memories of middle school and being blown across playgrounds by the famous Oklahoma winds, earning the nickname "feather." I was the new kid attempting to infiltrate cliques of lifelong friends. I was bright and shy, preferring reading over talking. My teeth were crooked and my knees knocked together when I walked. They did not know me, and my appearance did not meet criteria for them to *want* to know me.

My sense of my power and my individual voice were reflected in my small stature: I was quiet, meek, and afraid. At times, I even became invisible to others' eyes. Bullies only confirmed this, pointing out the ways in which I did not belong and how I was ultimately powerless. They compiled notes detailing how I was unworthy to be in their presence. Some went so far as to try choking me, to physically remove my voice. The message was clear: I, my body, and my voice were irrelevant to those around me.

As I got older, the sense of powerlessness was turned inward, and I began to blame my body as the source of the pain. Although I never spoke it aloud, it was deafening in my soul. The critic took over and soon I carried the bullies within me, embodying their derision. I had an overwhelming sense of not feeling at home in my own skin. When I tried to articulate it, all I could grasp was the hatred for my body. I felt I was not enough: not pretty enough, not curvy enough, not sexy enough. I longed for a day when I would look like the girls in the magazines, when others would think I was pretty. They seemed elegant, strong, and beautiful. I was thin, unsure, and maybe even looked as awkward as I felt.

Some responded by telling me to secure my beauty by addressing my physical shortcomings: make my arms more shapely by working out, become more alluring with lip gloss, or increase my charm by styling my hair. In this manner, I could attract the attention (read: approval) of boys. A friend vigilantly guarded me against developing an eating disorder. Rather than trying to "fix" the pain by reinforcing societal ideals, she shared education and statistics of the harm these ideals can bring. She was able to bear witness, teaching me the danger of turning on my own body. More importantly, she modeled an alternative by living powerfully in her own body—a body whose size did not meet societal demands. Bold, tenacious, and a phenomenal musician, she was, and is, unmistakably a force to be reckoned with.

Even though I did not go on to develop one myself, eating disorders resonated with me deeply. I started to notice a still small voice inside that connected with these ideas, with how one could develop an eating disorder. At their heart, these illnesses make you feel as if your voice has been surgically removed. They vilify the body, depicting it as the source of misery. They made sense, and a piece of me had found my purpose for helping others. For the first time I had a direction, yet I still felt lost, with more questions than answers.

# Running

I can't remember exactly when it was first suggested I give yoga a try. I ran from yoga (as hard as I could) for a really long time. Years, in fact. I was intimidated by what felt like rooms of hopelessly cool young, white women waiting to silence my voice. They were graceful, lithe, and confident. From the images in magazines to the DVD teachers, my awkward and klutzy body felt out of step from their mesmerizing practices. This was my earliest exposure to yoga culture: it seemed an exercise created only for the perfect elite, while I felt like the outcast looking in. All I knew of yoga was cool girls bending themselves into pretzels, ultimately becoming even more fabulous. I thought *of course* there was no way for me to fit into that category. Like a kinder, gentler bully, yoga excluded me as much as I ran from it.

Yet even as I ran, my yoga was there. I had moments of what could only be characterized as stillness and *being*—when there were no worries, the critic was silent, and I was fully at home. My yoga was there on cool summer nights with those who were the first to truly see me, windows rolled down, music turned up, driving with no destination in mind. In the memory of a boy in skinny jeans, consumed by the love we had and lost. It was there when we sang about uniting under the battle call of Johnny boy at the top of our lungs. It was there when nothing stood between us and our dreams but time. Those midnight drives taught me to question everything from the government's authority to my parents'. Those were the moments when I first began to realize I had a voice. Thanks to another strong, powerful woman, I shyly learned there was a possibility I could make my own choices and have my own thoughts, whether or not those around me agreed with them. But I was not ready. Seeing myself as inherently unworthy of it all, I ran from the chance to be *and* from myself.

Looking back, the pattern is clear: I had a habit of not only underestimating myself but also handing my power over to those around me. I valued my voice no more than those who tried to take it from me. I believed them. Every single one. I accepted it when they told me my voice sounded annoying, I was ugly, I was unworthy. I did not fight it. I ran. I ran in spite of these powerful women, who exposed me to feminism even before I knew it existed, who showed me the possibilities of living without fear, owning your truth, and living on your own terms. Although I hoped those possibilities could be true for me as well, I still was not ready to see that I already had what I needed.

But the truth is, I was not just running: I was searching. Having learned prior to this that I had no inherent value except for my appearance, I continued to look outside myself for validation. For someone, anyone, to truly see me: not my body, not my size, but me. Yet I was not ready to see myself. Whether it was attempting to capture the attention of some off-limits boy, getting into the right school, or generally finding approval, I simply could not see the possibilities I possessed. I was convinced I was both powerless and voiceless in spite of the enormous privilege I had been granted by society. I defined myself by what others saw in me. Being told multiple times that you are so small that "you don't take up any space" takes a toll. I felt angry, hurt, and scared as I shrunk even further into invisibility—in my own mind at least.

## Surrendering

My first yoga class, I was terrified. By this point I had spent a great deal of time reading about the philosophy of yoga, even going so far as to encourage others to give it a try and speak to its potential in treating eating disorders. Stepping into the studio for the first time, watching a line of graceful women stream out, I felt just like that gawky teenage girl yet again.

That all changed the second I stepped on the mat (okay, more like the second I stepped off the mat and could feel the effects of my practice). I felt different. Even in those first few practices, I bent and twisted my body in ways I not only thought I could not but had also been told I should not. In those poses, the poses I feared the most, I found my greatest freedom. I could feel myself coming into balance and alignment right along with my spine.

When you're on the mat, you can't run anymore. In fact, everything you run from will catch up with you and be acted out on the mat. Life out of sync? *Vrksasana* (tree pose) won't be happening today. Anxious and unsure? Forget *bakasana* (crow pose). Brain won't shut down? Good luck with *savasana* (corpse pose). The mat becomes your greatest classroom. On the mat, there is only you, your troubles, and your possibilities. Yoga forces you to live in your body with them. It forces you to see yourself, be yourself, and surrender to that truth. I am often struck by the still, quiet moments I once found on those midnight drives and have discovered they were not a fluke: they were the first moments of my life when I lived authentically and wholeheartedly. They were the first expression of my yoga, and I did not need asana to get there.

Yoga does not only force me to live in my body, it forces me to see me—all of me—for who I am. To do so, I had to give up the fight. I had to stop running. Here I was, waiting for the big reveal: the perfect kiss at the end of the fairy tale when I found my prince, the magnificent award in recognition of a long day at work, the light bulb going off. I was so busy searching, I never realized I was already there. I was always there, waiting to be noticed. Not by the world around me—not really. Their voices don't matter when it comes to my truth. I had to stop running; I had to stop fighting in order to find it. Only when I was able to let go, to surrender, was I finally able to arrive.

## Arriving

In coming home to my body, I am coming to know, understand, and finally realize my power—the good and the bad. To be honest, I often surprise myself with what I am able to do on the yoga mat if I stop shrinking away and living small—if I stop living the way the world sees me and begin living the way I am. So it is with my life.

This is the truth of who I am—all of me. I inhabit a thin, white body. I hit the jackpot not only genetically (giving me the body I have) but also in the experiences I was blessed to have. As a result, I am endowed with enormous unearned privilege in society. The simple fact of my body size means I am more likely to obtain a job, to find a romantic partner, to receive appropriate healthcare services, and to be able to live or breathe in public (or online) spaces without others expressing unfounded concern for my health and well-being.

In society, the act of living in a thin body means you are good, quiet, and obedient. You are appropriate, controlled, and always coloring within the lines. I took this persona on and accepted my privilege without question. I lived my life small and quiet, never speaking up, in spite of the fire growing inside of me for so long. In doing so, I harmed others with my silence and inaction. I have witnessed injustice and said nothing. I have been a racist, harming in my ignorance. I never realized the power I had to hurt others. By not speaking up, I allowed myself to become part of the problem.

Thin privilege may sound like the ultimate blessing, but the truth is that it harms women of all sizes. Although having this body gives me substantial power in society and makes my life easier in many ways, it also defines me by this single attribute. Thin privilege inherently limits my ability to be more and do more, because my worth is defined by my appearance. Those I systematically handed my power to over the years? They only saw the outside of me.

Society reduces all of us to its simplest, least offensive or challenging parts. The modern perception of yoga reduces it to an exotic workout. I am reduced to the part of my size, to being a thin woman whose only value is understood to be in her appearance. This is the least offensive part of me, as my size is inherently accepted by Western society. To be honest, I spent much of my life believing my worth was defined by external factors. I believed what others thought of me was absolute, and I remained ignorant of who I am at my core. It's likely I haven't changed at all, but have only grown to fully realize more and more of who I am and can be in this very moment. What I was seeking was already present within me, and was waiting only to be noticed and awakened.

In a similar fashion, the practice of yoga has shifted toward becoming an industry that has handed over much of the power for its true worth in favor of consumerism and monetary gain—the most tangible form of acceptance in contemporary society. Yoga culture, the face of yoga in society, teaches us that the practice is about bending over backward to touch our toes to our noses. In reality, the practice itself means many things to many different people. For some, yoga is a form of movement that keeps one limber and spry. For others, it is an expression of spirituality and meditation. Each of these individually is only a fraction of yoga. Yoga has the potential to be more than the sum of its parts. In its whole, yoga is a system for living, of which asana is only one piece. When taken together, it helps one find and maintain balance in their daily lives—something you will be acutely aware of when a single piece drops away even for a moment. The translation of the Sanskrit term *yoga* is simply "union"—the act of pursuing balance within and outside of yourself. For today, this is where I find my yoga practice: finding my edge physically, emotionally, and spiritually. Without it, my life quickly becomes out of sync.

Yoga helped me access my power, to appreciate my complexity, and to see the value of these things not just for myself but for others as well. Seeing myself as a whole person and finally realizing yoga as a whole practice has helped me understand that all things are not equal, but I have the power and the voice to do something about that. How would the stories of our time change if we were able to see yoga, see those around us, and even see ourselves as whole beings rather than bits and pieces? Imagine the possibilities if we let go of this reductionistic perspective of living that neglects the ultimate complexity and beauty of all beings, moving away from seeing characteristics and labels? What if we were able to see more than the outer shell of a person or being, and were instead able to appreciate the person, their experiences, and the greater culture this all exists within to create each unique being?

Even this understanding of yoga as an individual practice or pursuit of self-awareness is an act of living small. The very foundation of yoga has the power to address injustice and oppression when we as yogis, as a community, stop holding ourselves back with this perception. When we expand beyond our individual practices, yoga has the power to dramatically alter the world. We have the duty to act: to acknowledge our privilege, how it harms us and those around us, and to dismantle the systems of inequality. Only when we are able to see our power as it truly is and not allow society to use it to silence us can we truly be free.

Without question, the darkest moments in my life led to my greatest blessings. And I am only beginning to see the power I have. Although my previous motto was to play it safe by hiding inside a set of very well-developed armor, I ultimately created the biggest messes in my life by maintaining a facade that led others to perceive me as cold, angry, strong, and unapproachable. I now choose differently: to live my life bold, large, and authentic. The specific steps I have taken and the milestones I have reached along my journey are unimportant—truly. What *is* of vital importance is that my path, from the dark to the light and every bit in between, prepared me for this present moment. It empowered me with every skill, tenacious attribute, and driving force. The thin privilege I hold and the darkness I experienced have empowered me to have and use a voice where others may not. I intend to use that voice, to help others find their light.

My joy now lies in using my voice to end the war on women's bodies and the need for external approval to establish our worth. Far from silent, I advocate for size diversity. I work to draw attention to the complexities of power, autonomy, and integrity in society so that all may find freedom. My light drives me to target the deadliest mental illness of eating disorders (my day job). The gift of my yoga teacher training (my self-care and connection) saved me from a different darkness and empowered me to continue my own growth and participate in that of others'. I hope that my own experiences will allow me to create safe spaces for all students to participate in all that yoga can be and create opportunities for yoga teachers to deepen their awareness of their power to impact people on (and off) the mat. My vision, my hope, is for each one of us to be able to define our own journeys, write our own stories, and dictate where our power may lie.

The structures of privilege and oppression are insidious, so much so that they harm even those who they purport to benefit. We all suffer by virtue of the fact that we are not all free. It's time to listen, to hear our whole story. We decide where the power is, not the world. The choice is yours. Ask yourself: am I ready to stop living?

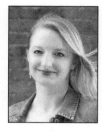

Jenny Copeland, PsyD, RYT, is a clinical psychologist with Ozark Center in southwest Missouri, specializing in the treatment of eating disorders. She strives to help people pursue balance within and outside themselves to find freedom in their bodies. Dr. Copeland is the cocreator of the Model of Appearance Perceptions and Stereotypes, and continues to write on the dynamics of power and privilege related to body size in hopes of creating safe spaces for all.

Author photo by Amelia Hill / Hill Creative.

# PART 1 MOVING INWARD & UPWARD

- What has influenced your body image?
- How would you describe the cultural standard of "beauty" or what is considered attractive for women and men? What do you notice about this norm? What is missing? What and who does it exclude?
- What characteristics or attributes are assigned to people who emulate the standard?
- What are the cultural costs of trying to live up to and/or not living up to this standard?
- How have you attempted to live up to the cultural standard of what is acceptable and desirable?
- Think of how we might change our definitions of beauty and worth.
- How has yoga and/or other mindfulness tools offered healing and self-acceptance?
- When have you felt the most comfortable with and in your body?
- If you haven't developed a yoga practice or explored other mindfulness tools, what has stopped you?
- Identify three ways you can practice compassion for yourself.
- Begin practicing at least one today.

# PART TWO

## *Healing the Body and Mind through Practice*

Moving into a place of wholeness, a state in which we reconnect and rediscover all parts of ourselves with compassion, forgiveness, and acceptance, is the outcome of deep healing work. Coming into that state of wholeness requires that we recognize and integrate all aspects of self—the mind, body, and spirit. For those growing up with the mind/body split as a key aspect of Western culture, this can pose challenges and contradict many of the cultural mantras we've taken for granted, such as "mind over matter" or "no pain, no gain." The former implies that the body is subject to our sheer will or mental desires and should submit. The latter reminds us that we should listen to the wants of the mind and silence the wisdom of the body.

Tiina Veer stumbled upon yoga as a mechanism to heal an injured body and discovered a physical practice that proved to be therapeutic. And while this is a gift in itself, there were deeper layers to this practice that bestowed gifts that are often overlooked. In fact, the physical practice has become the dominant focus in the North American "yoga scene" as well as the representation of yoga in most media imagery. It's no surprise, given the cultural obsession with the external form. But, if we look closer, as Veer did, yoga practice touches the heart and mind as well, providing new insights, perspectives, and emotional states of being. For Veer, this has resulted in unapologetic acceptance and contentment in a body that society often dismisses and condemns.

While feminism offered a form of empowerment, too often Beth Berila still felt the familiar pangs of guilt and judgment deep within her body. Her yoga practice offered newfound clarity and the ability to discern the messages and feelings that bubbled to the surface, allowing her to move into a deeper sense of authenticity coupled with compassion rather than judgment.

Kimber Simpkins invites us to discover and trust the expert within. Taught that a woman's thinness equated to her value, Simpkins spent much of her life dieting and absorbing the message that she could not be trusted around food. Thanks to continued yoga practice, Simpkins learned to trust the wisdom of her body and find a place of balance.

Addictions often go hand-in-hand. For Elena Brower, an addiction to control that manifested in both food restriction and drug addiction stemmed from deep wounds. Her story reminds us that each of our healing journeys have their own rhythm and timing—that they are far from linear or uniform in nature. In Brower's case, with time and patience, continued practice and the support and encouragement from a conscious community made all the difference.

For Dana Byerlee, yoga practice provided the foundation of a full-blown soul cleansing and rebirth. In an awe-inspiring and heartfelt narrative, she details her battle with breast cancer and the countless ways her yoga practice supported her ability to reevaluate, reconnect, and rejuvenate herself through the process.

Whereas yoga allowed Byerlee to battle cancer, yoga practice helped Jodi Strock battle an entirely different set of demons. A deepened disconnection to her body after she survived being raped in college led Strock to battle an eating disorder. Yoga was the mechanism to eventually allow her to reconnect with her body as well as develop compassion for her whole self, one composed of both shadow and light. As she explains, yoga continues to provide the space for healing, thereby allowing her to share her gifts with others.

# FINDING THE RIGHT FIT:
# A JOURNEY TO SELF-ACCEPTANCE

*by Tiina Veer*

Yoga has been one of the greatest gifts in my life. Coming to it in an abundant body and with invisible disabilities did, however, present unique challenges. Those challenges ended up being what inspired me to become a yoga teacher and, to this day, they continue to shape my practice and my teaching methodology and philosophy, and they continue to fuel my passion to help effect individual and social transformation through yoga.

## No Fat Chicks? Know Fat Chicks!

I'd been a massage therapist for several years by the time I decided I needed something to counterpoise the physical, repetitive nature of my work, to stay as pain free and functional as possible, and to have career longevity. I thought yoga would be perfect, offering more than an intelligent physical practice: there was meditation, philosophy, "spirituality"—one-stop shopping!

Assumptions about yoga being "all-embracing" were quickly dismantled. It was everything I thought it was *not* going to be. Judgy. Competitive. Inaccessible. Sometimes teachers completely ignored me, sometimes they inappropriately highlighted me, sometimes well-meaning teachers didn't have the skill or training to work effectively with my body (be it my size, my physical limitations, or both), sometimes it was how other students treated me, and there were entire studios that may as well have had "No Fat Chicks" signs hanging on their doors.

Many yoga texts say "yoga is a mirror to the Self." I came to realize that yoga is actually a mirror for *anything* it reflects—including our culture. Which is why many are now asking *"Why is there so little diversity in yoga spaces?"* It turns out the marginalization occurring in greater culture is mirrored in modern yoga culture as well—sizeism, racism, homophobia, ageism, ableism, healthism, all of it and more. Many of us are now attempting to dismantle this in our own worlds and collectively through organizations like the Yoga and Body Image Coalition.

## Mixed Feelings

My early yoga journey was tarnished by poor experiences, and I may very well have given up after a few classes if I hadn't fallen so deeply in love with the beauty and utility of the practice itself. In a city the size of Toronto, I knew I had to be able to find a space where I could feel comfortable and well met—little did I know that would take well over a year.

I was grateful to eventually find a couple of spaces where I felt comfortable (and one that used lots of props, a much rarer find back then), and it wasn't very long before I wanted to become a yoga teacher myself, specifically to fill the gap that I had experienced. I chose a lengthy teacher training not only because of the quality of the program, but because I wanted time to further develop my own practice before embarking on teaching. It was more than 700 hours held weekly over two years, which I completed and was then fortunate enough to attend again fully when I became anatomy faculty for the subsequent two-year group. It was an amazing four years of deepening into practice and self-inquiry. In the middle of it all, I founded Yoga for Round Bodies, and the rest is, as they say, history.

## Back to the Beginning

As a person of size, I am definitely affected in daily life by our strong cultural obsession with thinness and the implications of living large in a fat-hating society. Despite this, I have (miraculously) been able not to internalize these messages so deeply nor allow them a primary role in shaping my body or self-image. Yoga and, particularly, meditation have helped me to continually reinforce and refine this ongoing journey.

Despite being the lifetime owner/operator of a fat body, I grew up with pretty decent body image, in spite of the odds. Sometimes this alone has had me feel like a total and utter aberration. I've spent a lot of time thinking about how I managed to grow up fat (and female), and become a fat woman, and still have a relatively intact body image. A number of people, events, and even flukes stand out in forming an early base to a healthy body image, but perhaps none so much as something with roots in my ethnic heritage.

## Gettin' Naked

I was born in Canada but with parents and family from Estonia (a tiny northern Baltic nation). Being war survivors meant inherited trauma for me that would strongly affect self-image and mental health in other ways (depression, anxiety, irrational fear to name a few—all thankfully aided by yoga and therapy). But my body image was very positively underpinned by a specific aspect of Estonian culture—the communal sauna, a traditional bathing and social ritual.

Childhood to early adulthood, I spent oodles of time in saunas with my mother and many female family members and friends. From young to old; from thin to average to fat; short to tall; athletic to non-athletic; breasts low, breasts high; thin limbs, thick limbs; wrinkled skin, tight skin; round bellies, flat bellies; everything in between. Naked bodies as natural and normal as the sky and the earth. Unabashed. Unapologetic. Unflinching. Neither the topic of conversation nor the focus. An incredibly supportive beginning toward accepting my body as it was despite opposing external messages. From a young age, I got the idea that *it was just normal to have a body!* Which helped set the stage for a healthy body image. This points to a desperate need in our culture to normalize bodies—*all* bodies—so we can *all* heal from our collective body preoccupation.

## Mishaps, Mistreatment, then Massage Therapy

My inspiration to become a massage therapist was how it helped me to cope with chronic pain and injury. By nineteen, I'd been in four car accidents. First, at twelve. We were stopped when we were rear-ended at full speed by a driver who'd fallen asleep at the wheel, still drunk from the night before. I was in the front and the impact was so potent it broke my seat back. The first in a string of accidents leading to an altered body.

Then three more, one year after another, from seventeen to nineteen. Each with progressively worse tissue damage, each compounding injuries from the one before without ample time for healing in between. Especially after the third accident, I was experiencing chronic pain and occasionally "low back bouts" that would leave me on my back for weeks at a time, in severe pain, afraid to move.

At eighteen, another life-changing injury—downhill skiing, an activity I'd done with my family every winter weekend since I was six. I fell and my ski didn't release. My body went one way, my ski the other. I tore my anterior cruciate ligament (ACL).

The orthopaedic surgeon who attended me said I "was not an athlete, so wouldn't need the reparative surgery," and I was sent away with a script for physiotherapy. Months later, I was experiencing knee-locking. When I went back to the same doctor, he scoped my knee and found I'd also torn my medial meniscus. He removed the loose bodies, again sending me away with a script for physiotherapy.

I didn't know better then. He was a highly acclaimed expert, I had no reason to doubt his authority, or so I thought. I wouldn't become aware of the depth of weight stigma in medicine (and everywhere else) until later in life. On scoping my knee, he would have seen clearly how damaged my ACL actually was and a much later MRI with a different doctor revealed it was nearly severed. By then my knee was full of arthritis, too late for the reparative surgery that should have happened in the first place.

Regrettably, before that injury, even after the first two accidents, I was strong as an ox. But after years of having an unstable knee joint that affected my biomechanics, there are now multiple issues affecting my freedom of movement.

I'm left with an injured body that requires frequent micromanagement and can, at times, be a house of cards. Sometimes even small triggers can set me way back. I joke that massage therapy school was the best and most expensive "rehab" I did—it taught me how to manage my body issues, which gave me more freedom from pain (and allowed me to function at such a physical job).

I have to be careful trying new activities for fear of hurting myself and possibly creating yet another recovery period (not to mention potentially lost income). I even have to be careful about how long I walk, as hard flat surfaces like concrete do me in (which is why I adore hiking in the forest, it gives me more walking freedom plus the healing of nature). I go through periods of being able to exercise and move more assertively, but most of the time I need to stick with gentle and conservative practice to ensure I don't risk reinjury.

Possibly one of the most healing things I learned through yoga was to *never overpower my body,* even though this can unfortunately be a common theme in mainstream yoga—not necessarily with explicit instructions to "overpower" the body, but definitely with the common coachy direction or insinuation to go beyond one's perceived limits. Because of underlying fragility, I learned right from the get-go to look past this often regurgitated and unquestioned instruction and follow the wisdom of my body instead. What it asked for and needed was a gentle, moderate practice. Not ninja or Cirque du Soleil training. Perhaps some wish to explore "going beyond their limits" physically, but for me (and loads of others) this can be downright debilitating.

Looking at me, besides seeing a fat body—which some would consider a disability (I don't, I consider it a body size)—one would likely never know I suffer chronic pain and invisible disabilities that affect my life experience. I am under no illusions: I fully recognize that even with my invisible disabilities I still experience boatloads of able-bodied privilege (not to mention white privilege and other privileges) that allow me to move quite freely in the world. But it's yoga that helped me to accept my body's limitations and work with them, not against them. It has helped me accept the changeability of my body and not despair or grieve when "ground is lost," as inevitably happens from time to time. With a practice, there is hope that ground can be regained and tranquil acceptance when it cannot. This freedom from the expectation of *any* kind of "ideal body" is *extremely* liberating.

## Vector for Social Change

When I embark on telling my story of how yoga shifted my body acceptance, because of my size, it's often assumed that the story I will tell is one of coming to accept and love my abundance. Of course my roundness is a huge part of how I practice and experience yoga (and yoga culture), even how I offer my teaching—the truth is, though, the biggest impact of yoga on my body image was accepting my injuries and the reality of the limitations they created. It was liberating to let go of grieving the strong body I'd *once* had, and peacefully accept the body I *did* have, exactly as it was, limitations and all.

I started working on my body image relative to my size in my late twenties, on the back of the early experiences that helped me forge a positive relationship with my "flawed" body, *as society viewed it*. And that was the point. I realized then and before that I was not the problem. *It was society that was seriously messed up, not me.* If I hadn't already been working on that, I may never have had the courage to enter the healing field, become a massage therapist, and eventually end up here.

In a way, it was precisely from always having a very fat body that such acceptance could arise—I was so far outside the realm of society's take on an acceptable body, I had no choice but to love it (or at least accept it) or otherwise face a life of utter desperation and anguish. I decided I was not going to live my life like that.

This size acceptance is probably what saved me from chronic dieting too. I had come to accept my body as it was, so I could simply go about enjoying life the best I could, without feeling like I had to live on a perpetual diet to be "worthy." Ironically, ten years ago and well into my thirties, for the first time I started to feel pulled toward losing weight. Not so ironically, it was around the time that "obesity epidemic" rhetoric started really heating up in the media.

I tried three "healthy" attempts, each time losing weight, each time gaining it back and then some. I ended up forty pounds heavier than when I started dieting, with a loose and wobbly fat body in place of the taut fat body I previously occupied. And the worst outcome—slightly elevated blood pressure after a lifetime of running steady at the same numbers at the low end of healthy range. Fortunately, still within healthy range, but elevated nonetheless. It was obvious I needed to investigate what was going on before trying again and ending up gaining more weight.

At this time, already practicing yoga (and meditation since studying zen shiatsu), I was able to more readily come to terms with my new "less optimal" version 2.0 fat(ter) post-diet body. And zen and yoga philosophy had also been teaching me discernment: there is the illusion of truth and then there is truth.

So I started looking for answers and stumbled across information that shocked me so much it was like going down the rabbit hole in *Alice in Wonderland* or taking the red pill in *The Matrix*. I learned that much of what we think we know about weight and health is not actually evidence-based and rests tottering above an abyss of weight stigma. I was surprised to learn that 80 to 97 percent of intentional weight loss efforts fail long-term—within two to five years of starting a diet, the average dieter has regained all but about two pounds of the weight they lost, with anywhere from one- to two-thirds gaining more than was lost, leading to dangerous successions of loss and gain ("weight cycling"), correlated with all the things fatness is correlated with, and worse.

Wait a minute, *what??* So I *wasn't* an outlier? Regaining my weight and then some could have been pretty much *predicted?* On one hand, good news because it made me feel less like a failure, but it was *enraging!* To find out this information is known, even diet companies know (it's why they are mandated to put "results not typical" in all their advertising), and yet it's a failing and health-risking intervention still pushed like it's the Holy Grail, the answer to all ills.

Amid the depressing truth about weight loss, I thankfully stumbled upon the Health at Every Size® (HAES) paradigm, which is an evidence-based look at the conflation between weight and health and advocates a weight-neutral approach to individual health. It's often described as "the new peace movement for our bodies," and dovetailed beautifully with yoga philosophy and my practice.

By this point, I was also finding myself perpetually pissed for having gone down the weight loss path, and for all who have, are, and will inevitably go down it. Yoga and meditation not only gave me tools for staying even-keeled in the face of that anger but it also gave me a vector for creating social change, and it motivated me to advocate to end the "yoga for weight loss" trend, not only because it's unsubstantiated, but because it saddens me to see yoga used as a mule for the 60 billion dollar per year diet industrial complex.

I was just embarking on offering Yoga for Round Bodies training to teachers when I discovered both HAES and the size acceptance movement, immediately realizing the training wouldn't be complete without them. It was synchronicity. And now most of my offerings for teachers incorporate information on HAES, sizeism, and healthism (as well as exploring other types of marginalization and oppression—they all intersect).

I constantly encourage teachers to examine their own internalized weight stigma (almost impossible *not* to have in our size-obsessed culture), so they can do their best not to repeat stereotypes and micro-aggressions in class that larger-bodied people have to endure in almost every aspect of daily life. There is also self-healing that comes with ridding ourselves of internalized weight stigma—what do you think fuels our collective body-preoccupation, leading to a litany of problems not the least of which being life-threatening eating disorders?

## Yoga's Ultimate Gift

I entered yoga in an injured body looking to heal it, so I've always had to be moderate and careful when approaching asana. I was never particularly interested in practicing like a ninja, acrobat, nor dancer, nor having yet another new thing at which to excel. I just wanted to function and heal and have a practice that supported peacefulness and more comfortable everyday living.

Like most everyone else, my challenge was to accept my body and myself exactly as they were, messiness included. For me, this meant fully accepting my so-called flaws, especially my limitations. I often had to fight that opposing message so common in yoga classes about not accepting our "perceived limitations." I had to carefully discern the difference. And though I was savvy enough not to try to constantly push through my limitations, I still had loads to learn about quieting my constant desire for them to be different—such an unnecessary mental and emotional strain.

Yoga asana gives me a physical practice that is truly therapeutic and can meet my constantly-changing body. It challenges me to fully accept my body, especially when I'm feeling down on function and what's possible (for example, there have been periods of time where all that was doable was Restorative practice, and instead of lamenting that I couldn't do more, I appreciated that I still had a practice). This ever-shifting practice allows me to focus on (and appreciate) what my body does for me, what it can do instead of what it can't, and above all, that it still functions as the awe-inspiring spaceship that allows me to have this earthly experience. Everything else is window dressing.

Asana and meditation have taught me so much about comparative mind consistently undermining our potential to experience contentment, which I believe rests at the heart of experiencing true happiness. It has given me tools to use for personal transformation and daily self-care, and even to effect social change. Yoga has truly come to perfume every corner of my life, and is slowly but surely working to help me attain a lofty goal: finding contentment and becoming unflappable.

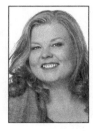

Tiina Veer founded Yoga for Round Bodies™ in 2004. A pioneer in the accessible yoga movement, she has trained teachers all over the world how to sensitively teach bigger-bodied yogis, apprehensive beginners, and those with chronic pain or injury. She is a veteran manual therapist, founder of Halcyon Health Wellness Centre in Toronto, Canada, and an avid advocate of the Size Acceptance movement and Health at Every Size® paradigm. Veer is most passionate about simple self-care and empowering people to become the source of their own guidance and inspiration. www.tiinaveer.com

Author photo by Donna Santos.

# SPARKLE GIRL

## *Dr. Beth Berila*

A friend of mine calls me Sparkle Girl. She used it to describe how I learned, early in my childhood, to please others and to gain my self-worth through external approval. My family says that I used to come home from preschool crying and apologizing for getting my dress dirty. They never understood where I learned that I was supposed to be spotless and perfect, since they never cared whether my dress was dirty from playing. But, somehow, I had already absorbed those messages, constantly worried about other people's judgment of me, certain I wasn't good enough.

The cultural patterns in the media, my schooling, my family, and my community told me that if I was the "good little girl" I would get approval and be loved. Since I wasn't traditionally pretty, being "good" meant being smart and caretaking. It was my unspoken role in the family to take care of other people's emotions. To this day, I have to resist the tendency to be more aware of other people's states of being than my own. Until I found yoga many years later, I often lived more in my mind than in my body, seeing myself through the eyes of others.

One day, probably in my sophomore year of high school, I set myself the goal of being valedictorian. One might admire the determination to achieve high standards, except the real motivation was to prove my worth. I was certain that once I achieved it, people would finally see me, and I could truly be myself. For years I strived for that goal, giving myself migraines, panic attacks, and depression, until I was finally named co-valedictorian. While my family was proud of me, it was a rather empty achievement. As with many of the external accolades I tried to earn to validate myself, they never worked. I wouldn't understand why until I found feminism, then yoga, then learned to integrate the two into a deeply healing way of being.

Though I lived a very privileged and loving childhood, I deeply absorbed the sexist messages in the culture. Those messages told me that my worth as a girl and woman depended on people's approval of me. They were amplified by the sense that something was wrong with me because of my queerness, though I wouldn't discover that until my midtwenties. To use psychologist Beverly Tatum's metaphor, I breathed in the oppressive beliefs like I would smog, and it tainted how I saw myself and the world.[1]

Eventually, feminism would teach me that this is called internalized oppression, and here's how it works: negative messages about women, people of color, LGBTQ+ folks, and other marginalized groups saturate US culture. Authentic, positive narratives about these communities are rare. So we begin to accept those beliefs about ourselves and others like us. We absorb them for so long and often over so many generations that these harmful messages erode our very identities. *We begin telling them to ourselves*, participating in our own oppression from within. Unless we can counter them with some empowering messages about our group, it is virtually impossible to unearth these toxic beliefs and come to a holistic, empowered sense of self.

## Can Feminists Sparkle?

When I went to college, I found feminism and my world transformed. I took several courses on the feminization of poverty from the resident Marxist Feminist economics professor who rocked my world. The first actual Women's Studies course I took was called "Decolonizing Femi-

1. Beverly Tatum, "Defining Racism: Can We Talk?" in *Women: Images and Realities, A Multicultural Anthology*, 4th ed., eds. Amy Kesselman, Lily D. McNair, and Nancy Schiedewind (NY: McGraw-Hill, 2006), 386–390.

nisms." We read Chandra Talpade Mohanty while watching the Anita Hill and Clarence Thomas televised hearings. I finally had a language to explain the worldview that had long lingered at the edges of my consciousness. My awareness of deep injustice grew exponentially. I voraciously read the fiction of women of color and informed myself about the oppression of marginalized groups. I was empowered, I was righteous, and I was passionate.

This feminist empowerment continued through my masters program and into my doctorate, where I became a Women's Studies teaching assistant and completed a dissertation in community-based arts as a form of feminist social change. The central New York town where I earned my doctorate was also a hotbed of community activism, and I learned a great deal about community organizing. I came out as a lesbian during that time and stepped right into participation in the transmenace direct action group for transgender justice. I felt empowered and informed. I spoke out about injustice and educated myself and others about feminist social change.

## Unlearning Internal Oppression

It was during my doctoral program that I discovered yoga. I was drawn to its promise of wholeness and peace, but for many years I could only sip its potential. I practiced with an Anusara (Hatha yoga) teacher, which hooked me because its emphasis on anatomy focused my attention on my embodied experience. I also loved that it helped me take the yogic insights to my life off the mat. But as hungry as I was for all of that, I couldn't hold it. When I returned to my graduate work, I would quickly resume the life of the (judgmental) mind.

While I advocated for feminist empowerment, the ability to see power and oppression too often morphed into yet another way to beat myself up. Rather than accepting mistakes in unlearning privilege as a part of the process, these missteps convinced me that I was an awful feminist. This was more than the proverbial white guilt, because it was also a familiar, old narrative. It *felt* familiar in my body. One minute I would be righteously pointing out inequality, but the next, I would see a complexity that I had missed and that familiar voice of judgment would erupt again. I would disassociate, flush, and my body would contract. I would either want to run away or ramp up the perfectionism. Neither resulted in social justice or healing.

This judgment was intensified by graduate school, where we were taught to find the flaws in someone else's argument before we looked for the contributions. We learned to tear down without necessarily bothering to create new, empowering alternatives. For someone who had internalized sexist and homophobic messages so deeply that I determined my self-worth by external approval, these patterns intensified one another.

The result was profound feminist strength that was consistently undermined by invalidating self-talk. Even as I write this, here is the external and internal monologue that is going on:

**External:** *Sexist messages so pervade our culture that I learned, from a young age, that my self-worth is based on external approval and the degree to which I make other people happy. Feminism, while empowering, also intensified that internal critique, sometimes further demoralizing my already weak sense of self.*

**Internal Story Line:** *How full of yourself are you? Honestly, people in the world have REAL oppression—Syrian refugees who are barely surviving on rafts while fleeing horrendous violence, transyouth of color who are being murdered throughout the world, and many women of color who don't get the luxury of this white, middle class, pityfest that you are having right now.*

This cacophony played havoc with my sense of self for years. There is some truth to the critique in the internal narrative. The version of sexism and homophobia that I absorbed was indeed a white, middle class one. It is NOT the lived oppression that many marginalized groups face, which is, arguably, much more tangibly violent. That is the feminist wisdom of the internal monologue above. However, the shaming and dismissive tone in which it is delivered gets in the way of that wisdom. I wouldn't learn to discern the difference until well into my thirties.

Several years later, after earning tenure, I returned to yoga. My heart and body told me that I needed healing or else. So I completed a 200-

hour teacher training with Senior Anusara instructors. I delved deeper and deeper into my own practice and eventually completed a 340-hour teacher training in Tantric yoga and Ayurveda. Finally, I began to touch that deep yogic insight. I learned to listen for the inner voice that is filled with loving-kindness and acceptance. I began to discern that this voice is more expansive than the harmful messages. It helps me unearth them with fierce compassion, which the Buddhist teacher Sharon Salzburg defines as, "a potent tool for transformation since it requires us to step outside of our conditioned response patterns." [2]

Through my yoga practice, I have reflected very carefully on which parts of those inner monologues are socialized privilege that I have to unlearn and which parts are internalized oppression that I also have to unlearn. The line between the two is not always clear. But here is what I do know. While there is often some deep wisdom in these inner monologues, that insight is drowned out by the harsh shaming. What distinguishes the two is tone and effect: wisdom opens up possibility and resonates as truth in my gut. Internalized oppression demoralizes and demeans.

Yoga and meditation helped me reconnect to my body and begin to distinguish between embodied wisdom and toxic messages. They *feel* dramatically different. I now lead workshops on yoga and meditation for unlearning internalized oppression. Participants consistently say similar things. Internalized oppression, when it strikes, makes us feel small, threatened, and unsafe. We disassociate. Our hearts race. We break out in sweat. We flush. We want to hide. While different identity groups likely experience it in different ways, we can generally *feel* that something is wrong. Even if we believe the harmful messages, they do not sit well in our bodies and hearts. When we tap into authentic inner wisdom, on the other hand, it is not judgmental or invalidating. Even if it guides us toward change, it does so with compassion and a certainty of our worth.

---

2. Sharon Salzburg, "Fierce Compassion," *Huffington Post*, August 14, 2012, Accessed December 26, 2015, http://www.huffingtonpost.com/sharon-salzberg/fierce-compassion_b_1775414.html.

Instead of allowing room for *both* the privilege and the internalized oppression—which would then allow me to dismantle BOTH—the demoralizing messages let me know, in no uncertain terms, that my experiences and feelings do not matter. And that, I think, is a deeply un-feminist and nonyogic message. Rather than leading one to a deeper authenticity and connection with other people, this message becomes yet another tool to bludgeon oneself into submission. The shaming devaluation of one's own story is a tool of oppression. As the Chicana feminist Cherríe Moraga wrote, "If we are interested in building a movement that will not constantly be subverted by internal differences, then we must build from the inside out, not the other way around. Coming to terms with the suffering of others has never meant looking away from our own."[3]

## Yoga As a Path to My Inner Sparkle

My yoga practice kept coaxing me toward a wholeness that I longed for. It kept showing me signs that my feminism could be more empowering and holistic, if I could become embodied and unlearn those toxic messages. It helped me see that turning toward the pain, reflecting on it, and moving through it would help me heal. My practice helped me learn how to sit with discomfort and make more intentional choices about how to respond to it.

But, as empowering as yoga was, it also felt restricted at times, especially when I felt pressured to shut off any social critique in yogic spaces. Though many of the people with whom I have practiced over the years would probably identify as liberal, feminist analysis about the yoga spaces themselves was often unwelcome. Raising questions about cultural appropriation, challenging racial exclusions, or calling out the economic inaccessibility of many programs were not popular topics.

---

3. Cherríe Moraga, "Refugees of a World on Fire: Foreword to Second Edition," *This Bridge Called My Back: Writings By Radical Women of Color*, eds. Cherríe Moraga, Gloria Anzaldua ; foreword, Toni Cade Bambara (New York: Kitchen Table Women of Color Press, 1983), iii. Accessed December 26, 2015. http://monoskop.org/images/e/e2/Moraga_Cherrie_Anzaldual_Gloria_eds_This_Bridge_Called_My_Back_Writings_by_Radical_Women_of_Color-Kitchen_Table_Women_of_Color_Press.pdf.

They were often shut down with the message that these spaces were for "peace" not debate.

As a Women's Studies professor, I am no stranger to taking unpopular stances or to challenging people to reflect on their privilege when they don't want to do so. But it is disheartening in spaces that profess to be about liberation. It is painful to hear language of personal reflection and transformation, and then see yogis refuse to engage power and privilege around race, queerness, class, gender, or dis/ability.

## Reclaiming the Sparkle: Cultivating Discernment on the Mat

Once I deepened my yoga practice, the inner critique would still happen, but it would be tempered by what one of my yoga teachers calls "the holy pause" that would keep me from traveling down the reactionary path before I even knew I was having reaction. My inner monologue would then look something like this:

**Internal Story Line** (said in a shaming, harsh tone): *So you think you are a feminist change agent? Great. Why are you practicing yoga instead of doing social change?* Pause. Breathe. Step back to downward dog. Turn inward. Soften. (Shaming voice resumes, now a few decibels quieter.) *Do you know how many people can't afford yoga, or don't have the leisure time in their loves for yuppie "self-care" efforts because they have to work? The very fact that you are here means you are embracing your privilege—your class privilege and your white privilege (I mean really, do you see any people of color in this yoga studio)?"* Ujjayi breathing, connect with my heart. Hear the wisdom but not the shaming. Imagine sending kindness and compassion into my heart, connecting with that which is already there. What does my inner wisdom have to say? (Now even quieter.) *You should really be out there doing more ... you are an imposter ...* Breathe, deepen, connect ..." This is the story line. The one you have learned. Don't feed it. Soften your heart.

The ability to cultivate this discernment on my mat translated to much more skillful practice off my mat. I started moving in the world with much more heart-centered energy and skillful discernment. This wasn't a flawless process, of course, but yoga taught me that even the missteps were opportunities for transformation.

Eventually, I found my people: people who are, like me, integrating yoga and feminism in social justice work both on and off the mat. Organizations such as Off the Mat into the World, Yoga for All, and the Yoga and Body Image Coalition are spearheading some of this change. Studios are offering classes specifically geared toward supporting marginalized groups, including Queer and Trans Yoga, Accessible Yoga, and People of Colour Yoga. Moreover, a growing number of academics, myself included, are integrating feminism, yoga, social justice, and mindfulness, reflecting on both the possibilities of those partnerships and their limitations. These conversations mean that I no longer need to separate parts of myself. Yoga has helped me see that it is not really possible for me to separate those parts of myself and really show up to do good social justice work. Social justice movements need all of me. All of us.

Now when I come to my mat the story lines show up far less often. They are no longer the baseline. But when they do appear, they sound more like this:

**Internal Story Line:** (at a much lower volume, a much gentler tone of voice): *You should really be doing more.* You are doing what you can. *Self-care is for the pampered and privileged.* If you don't care for yourself, you cannot do the work for the long haul, nor can you do it skillfully. Sink into your body. Feel how this downward dog feels in your back, in your neck, in your heart center. Breathe into that connection with your heart. Feel the breath link your mind and your heart, letting the mind be a partner rather than dominate your heart. These messages that you are never enough ... they are learned messages. They can be unlearned. Breathe. Sink into your felt sense. Connect to your heart.

Until it is no longer just an inner monologue but rather an integrated sense of being. My whole self, as I am. Both my feminism and my yoga are practices in which the mistakes are as rich as any successes because of what they help me learn about myself, my role in oppressive systems, and my participation in liberation. On this journey, the inquiry has become: *What does your inner wisdom, informed by both your feminism*

and your yoga, guide you to say, do, or be in this moment? What is your embodied wisdom? Extend that to your relations to others in your community. Your
sparkle is your gift. Not a show to put on to please others ... you are already
worthy. Your sparkle is the unique light that each of us has to contribute to the
world. Claim it. Celebrate it. Use it to fuel your social change work. Sparkle on.
Hold here.

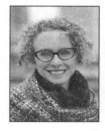

Beth Berila, PhD, 500-hr RYT, is the director of the
Women's Studies Program and professor in the Ethnic
and Women's Studies Department at St. Cloud State
University in St. Cloud, Minnesota. She is also a 500-
hour registered yoga teacher and an Ayurvedic Yoga
Specialist who completed her 500-hour Yoga Teacher
Training program at Devanadi School of Yoga and
Wellness. She is the author of the book *Integrating
Mindfulness into Anti-Oppression Pedagogy: Social Justice
in Higher Education* (Routledge). She served on the
leadership team of the Yoga and Body Image Coalition for two years and is now a community partner.
Her current projects merge yoga and meditation practices with feminism and mindful education to create a
form of socially engaged embodied learning.

Author photo by Haley Friesen.

# THE EXPERT WITHIN

## *Kimber Simpkins*

Our group of sweaty, tired trainees sank into the final *savasana* of the weekend as our yoga teacher trainer quoted Erich Schiffmann's invitation to trust ourselves without reservation. Despite my exhaustion, my mind perked up as I lay under the heavy blanket. Was it really true—could I just listen to my body and heart and they would unfailingly tell me what to do? Could I learn to trust myself that deeply?

It was easy to see how listening to myself applied to my yoga practice: I'd noticed that no matter how many times I did headstand, with any teacher, with perfect alignment, I eventually tweaked my neck. My body was telling me that headstand, the king of the asanas, was not majestic for me. I noticed my gut instincts about whether someone I'd met would return my phone call were surprisingly reliable—except when my enthusiasm for wanting to know the person better overruled my belly's quiet counsel. My trust in myself led me to quit my life as a lawyer and seek out a more family friendly and heart-true path, but I didn't know if it could help me come to grips with the one thing that dominated my whole life: food.

## Stuck Between Good and Bad

Ever since I struggled with disordered eating at age fifteen, I'd been hungry, and not because there weren't plenty of homemade grilled cheese sandwiches to go around. Hunger arose out of my ability to dissect and calculate the nutritional value of every edible item on my plate to the twenty-third decimal place and then to deprive myself of anything over my stingy calorie allotment. My body lodged its complaints with growling and shakiness, which I struggled all day to ignore. Was it a "good" day? Did I eat few enough calories? Or a "bad" day ... when my hunger raced passed the finish line of my diet? Had I eaten "good" food or "bad" food? If apples—which were supposedly "good" for you—had around 90 calories, and this diet cereal bar had only 75 calories and more vitamins, wasn't it "better" for me to eat the packaged thing? No. Yes. No. If I ate "good" foods during the day, I was "good." If I ate "bad" foods, no matter how many things I accomplished or checked off my to-do list, I was "bad."

Since my first diet at age twelve, I learned alongside my mom that there was no such thing as being "too thin," and that even women who looked fine to me might be called "fat," which seemed to also mean "bad" and "unworthy." I wanted to be worthy. I wanted to be good. And if eating as little as possible was the route to putting "bad" in the rearview mirror, I would press on the acceleration pedal and eat as little as possible. Dieting was the map to Worthy Body Land. Whenever one diet ran out of gas, I searched for another one, hopefully faster and better.

Well into my twenties, my mind churned with a dozen different diet experts' opinions about what was and wasn't good for me, and of course they couldn't agree among themselves on what was healthy or not. As a newly minted yoga teacher, I tried to eat "well"—a vegetarian diet with salads and fruit every day—but would frequently find myself mindlessly consuming entire bags of Cheetos or a box of drugstore chocolates.

"Chocolates are vegetarian," I consoled myself.

I did not trust myself around cake. Or candy. Or bread. Or chips. I didn't trust myself around food. Period. I might eat "bad" foods until my stomach hurt one day, and eat "good" foods to the same painful threshold the next. I hated being caught up in the duality of good/bad, healthy/unhealthy, worthy/unworthy, but my brain rewarded a green smoothie with a big yogic gold star and French fries as an embarrassing failure of self-discipline. Even though yoga was all about bringing opposites into balanced relationship with each other, I found myself swinging on a pendulum of self-hatred on one side and smugness on the other, leaving any equanimity far behind.

What if I accepted Erich Schiffman's yogic invitation to trust myself? From my practice I knew my body was smart; wise in telling me when to let my wrists rest from too much arm balancing, insightful in knowing my hamstrings could safely stretch a little further in a forward bend, and tender in reminding me to rest, even in the middle of my practice, when the day's energy had run out with hours still left on the clock.

What if I radically embraced the possibility that my body knew what to feed itself, knew what belonged on its plate, in its mouth, and in its belly? What if I rejected the ideas of "good" and "bad" food and instead let my body find its way to moderation and enjoyment? Perhaps out of all the experts in the world, I'd been ignoring the one I should have been listening to all along: my own body.

Fear snuck in around giving up the expert's ideas of "good" and "bad." *What if I gain weight ... or lose weight? What if I get sick ... or get well?* I didn't know. But I did know that what I was doing—listening to everyone but myself—wasn't working.

I jumped. I took a leap of faith like I'd never taken before, and my body caught me. I'd always heard stories of those mystical people who could savor one bitty piece of chocolate a day and not finish a whole bar for weeks. From my own experience of the hamster wheel of binging and deprivation, I figured those people were masters of an iron-clad willpower that had deserted me long ago.

But my body taught me how to join their magical ranks. And upon my arrival it all made sense. There's no willpower. There's only listening to that clear, compassionate inner directive.

I had to bring the same principles I'd learned from stretching on my mat to sitting at the table: listen, trust, respond, feel. Listen to whether I was hungry or full, and to what I was hungry for. Trust my body's signals and enjoyment. Respond to what it's asking for and feel what's happening in my body moment to moment. I dumped all the ideas about what I could and couldn't do, what was allegedly "good" for me and "bad" for me, what I was supposed to do and not supposed to do, and let my body lead the way, the same way I would if I was taking my body into a difficult pose. I had to treat my body like it was the expert instead of all the diet gurus I'd carried around with me in my head.

Our tendency to divide food into good/bad categories isn't self-made. We tend to put a lot of faith in the "cult of the expert": where we look to someone with degrees, experience, or fame to tell us what we should or shouldn't do. Sometimes their information is appropriate and accurate and sometimes not. The problem is that we tend to believe experts over our own experience, substituting their advice in place of the experience of listening to ourselves and tuning in to what is right for us. We do this when we take on a new diet … first buying into the belief that thinner is better and healthier, and then that someone else has the secret to what our body should or shouldn't eat in order to make it look the way we want. And out of our fear and longing, we pour money into the pockets of the diet industry—more than 61 billion dollars a year. Even worse, with the 95-percent failure rate of weight loss diets,[1] the vast majority of the time we end up right back where we started, with an extra serving of self-hatred on the side, still convinced it's our own fault for not finding the right expert and the right diet.

Buddha told his followers to not simply believe him, but to try out the teachings themselves and see if his guidance tested true in the crucible of their own experience. I've heard many teachers repeat this same sentiment in yoga class: there's no requirement that you believe any particular dogma or doctrine in yoga. You only have to believe what you've experienced in your own mind, body, and heart. But in our scarcity-based culture it becomes very tempting to claim to have or know all the

---

1. DM Garner and S. Wooley, "Confronting the failure of behavioral and dietary treatments for obesity" *Clinical Psychology Review* (1991): 11:729–780.

answers, and sell books or workshops or programs to hungry people seeking those answers.

When I was one of those hungry people, I went looking for experts to show me how to feel full after and between meals, as well as how to treat my body with more love. Ayurveda, the traditionally Indian form of medicine, sounded intriguing, and I found an Ayurvedic cleanse offered at my local yoga studio. Many aspects of the cleanse were satisfying: I loved kitchari, the traditional curried lentil and rice stew eaten every day; massaging my body every day with sesame oil was magical; adding ghee (clarified butter) to my cooking made my life better; and water soaked almonds turned out to be a yummy treat I still savor. The practices I learned supported my concerted effort to listen to my body's needs and pay attention to what it wanted and enjoyed. Our workshop leader phrased everything as an invitation, allowing us to try things out and see how they felt in our bodies.

But when I opened a book a friend recommended about Ayurveda, it was full of lists of "don't eat this, eat this" and "this food is terrible for you, but this food is good for you." Things that my body loved—avocados and popcorn—were suddenly on the "bad" list. I shut the book and put it away. Nothing like a list of dos and don'ts to trigger my old eating disorder mind-set.

Looking around my yoga community, I saw that following seemingly "healthy" vegan, gluten-free, or other diets could turn otherwise rational humans into obsessive debators of "clean" versus "junky" food, the near enemies of my dearly departed "good"/"bad" dichotomy. The desire to eat well and take care of our bodies can take a destructive turn when we stop listening to what our bodies need and instead listen to some idea in our heads about eating only organic, sustainable, fairtrade, free-range, angel-grown foods. A term has been coined for this newish eating disorder—orthorexia—where one feels the need to eat "better" than others, strives for an ideal purity of the body, and ends up depriving the body of essential nutrients. Unfortunately, orthorexia is a sad direction our yoga practice can take us in if we ignore the body's needs and wisdom in favor of abstract ideas of purity and perfection.

We seldom like to acknowledge it, but yoga can be used to heal or to harm ourselves.

To finally exorcise the ghost of my eating disorder, I had to resolve to stop treating food like grace and sin, reward and punishment. I had to let food just be food, and learn that eating food, whatever its nutritional qualities or quantities, should not be an excuse for self-flagellation, denial, or even a feeling of lofty superiority. Just like how I was learning to treat my body on my mat, my meals needed more equanimity and mindfulness and less judgment and fear.

## Body Shame on the Mat

As healing as yoga was for my body and mind, I also found myself sometimes triggered by teachers around my eating disorder during yoga classes. One Tuesday night found me in class with a young teacher I knew from my training, who led fun, energetic classes. The lights were low and the room warm: my body was already looking forward to *savasana*. We were all in pigeon pose, bowed over the front edge of our mats when I heard her say:

"What am I going to do about these thighs?"

Did my teacher really just say that? Out loud? I wondered if my inner critic had parachuted out of my ear and climbed up into her mouth. And wait … if she thinks there's something wrong with her thighs … what does she think about mine?

*Her body's beautiful,* I thought. *I wish I looked like her.*

And suddenly the practice I found so comforting felt unsafe. Her comment awakened the old voices that told me I wasn't good enough. Heading home after class, I reminded myself that she didn't usually say that kind of thing and that she probably didn't mean it the way it sounded. Maybe I'd missed the context somehow? Most of her teaching was about accepting yourself as you are, so she must have had an off night. I was trying to talk myself down. I didn't want to give up an otherwise wonderful class.

Since I'd begun my yoga practice, I found spreading my toes on my mat to be an incredible way to reconnect with my body after years bent over law school textbooks. Before yoga, I had basically ignored my body until it started screaming at me in the only language I listened to: immobilizing back pain. On my mat, one teacher showed me how strong and flexible my body was. Another showed me how to do handstand, a superpower I'd never gotten the hang of as a kid. Another teacher showed me that I wasn't breathing into my back body at all ... wait, I have a back body? I found muscles on my side waist that I never knew were there, sore for the first time from twisting poses. I patiently learned to open my hamstrings and let my fingertips reach the earth—without reinjuring my back.

Yoga helped me find balance and notice where my body was in space ... resulting in fewer pratfalls and bruised knees from what I had always felt was a subtle hostility directed at me by the sidewalk. Slowly yoga was teaching me to trust my body and know that I could depend on its deep strength and wisdom. The message seeped in a little bit with every breath: I didn't need to wage war against my body. The teachings on compassion even gave me hope that I could make friends with it and see the good in this warm, alive being I inhabit.

Almost all the messages I heard in yoga were body affirming: supporting and inspiring a sense of peace and well-being in me and toward my body. Almost all.

Recalling my teacher's gaffe, I realized it wasn't the first time I'd been triggered by diet talk or body shaming around her. I'd heard her talk about being on charcoal and clay cleanses, which sounded like drastic diets. From other teachers I'd heard comments like, "Today, we're going to work off all those holiday treats," or "Five more times for that extra slice of pizza you had last night." Once in a room full of two hundred yogis, I heard the teacher punctuate a student's demonstration of a difficult pose with, "And that's why you keep off those extra five pounds."

It's an inconsistency for sure. On one hand the yoga teachings echoed loud and clear: you and your body are good, whole, wise, and don't need fixing. On the other hand, the same body-shaming language I'd heard from gym teachers and aerobics instructors and softball coaches who thought they were military sergeants sometimes crept into the instructions of how to engage your thigh muscles and draw your shoulders back. This inconsistency stretches back to the very roots of yoga. In fact, the hatha yoga we practice today arose in part out of the desire to perfect the human body (and spirit) and achieve immortality. The impulse to learn from an expert how to perfect the body has been part of the yoga tradition for centuries.

This contradiction is embedded in many traditions: seeing wisdom and divinity within each individual versus constraining all wisdom and divinity solely within the priests, texts, and icons. Throughout yoga history and throughout the history of many traditions, conflicts have arisen between institutional religions that reserve divinity and their more mystical counterparts. It's the belief structure version of dictatorship versus democracy: putting the power of feeling connected to the divine into the hands of one versus recognizing that power in everyone.

We see this in yoga class when a teacher takes power away from the students with statements like "I can show you the way. I know the truth. Listen to me. All the teachings come through me. If you want to perfect yourself, follow me." It gives power back to the students for the teacher to say "The truth is you already know the way. Everything you need to know is already in your heart. Listen to your heart and body. Let any teachings you hear help you move closer to yourself. You are already perfect. Follow the wisdom of your own heart." Many yoga teachers end up sharing a mixture of both of these messages, intentionally or unintentionally.

There can be real wisdom in listening to the "expert" and then trying things out to see how your body—the true expert—responds. It's the role of the teacher to take what they've heard from experts and teachings and offer the best to their students and let the real expert of their own bodies decide. Every body is different and responds differently to different foods and exercise and experiences. Our role as alive beings in sensitive animal bodies is to listen to those bodies, to pay attention to what they have to tell us over long years of growing and changing, and even observe the effects of billions of years of evolution on our bodies and hearts.

As students we must know that our teachers are imperfect and struggle with the same difficulties we do. We must be aware that while yoga practice can tend the seeds of healing, it can also water the seeds of self-cruelty and forgetting to listen to our own wisdom. When I go to yoga class nowadays I like to check in with my expert-in-residence. Does my body feel safe in this space and trusted by the teacher? If yes, then I let my body's enjoyment lead the way. The inner voice that reminds you that your body is trustworthy is the true expert within. You'll never regret finding teachers and classes that remind you over and over to listen to your loving internal guidance.

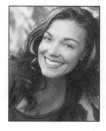

Kimber Simpkins is a longtime yoga instructor in the San Francisco Bay Area, body image coach, and the author of *Full* and *52 Ways to Love Your Body*. Her journey from private body hating to public body loving has inspired students and readers all over the world. Find out more at kimberyoga.com.

Author photo by In Her Image Photography.

# EVOLVING ADDICTION

## *Elena Brower*

Standing on my roof, squinting my eyes on that last bright day, reality hit me. The sun shone on the East River, the October air was the perfect crispness in New York City, and I was thirty-two floors up, praying. Praying for freedom. Praying for peace. Praying to be released from this prison of my own design, from this prison of addiction that I'd built around myself thirty years prior.

I was praying that I could do what I knew I finally needed to do. Praying in my heart and soul that this was the end of the road. That I would not be getting high again, I would not be hurting myself again, and I would not be spending any more time hiding and lying again. I was ready for the end, and I felt the burgeoning beginning of significant shift. I was ready to grow up. I'd just turned forty-five two weeks prior.

My relationship with addiction began when I was fifteen. I'd begun hanging around with a bunch of older kids, mostly seventeen-year-olds, who were "popular" pot smokers, who made life seem far more interesting than I'd ever imagined. Soon my grades deteriorated, but I knew I wanted to go to a great university, so I figured out how to maintain my grades and keep on partying.

Around that time was the first time I've ever smoked a cigarette; an unforgettable afternoon in a tree house with my unconditional best friends, and we must've smoked an entire pack of Parliament Lights. We laughed, we stunk, and we managed to keep that secret for a long while. After emerging from a childhood of endless car rides during which the elders in the car would smoke (and we'd cough, complain, whine, and moan to PLEASE open the window a bit more), smoking suddenly became sexy, and I was hooked.

I'd sneak cigarettes in the bathroom at home, blowing smoke into the ceiling vent, saved by the fact that both parents smoked so it was relatively undetectable. I loved the look of my hand holding the cigarette—it reminded me of my mom's hand out the car window, during those moments when she seemed most calm, whether she was driving or standing out in our backyard taking some time to herself. I was growing up and I loved the feeling of autonomy that smoking seemed to bring me.

While I'd quit several times over the course of the next three decades, tobacco and marijuana were simultaneously my salvation and my prison. At times I could convince myself that my most treasured moments of release were accompanied by both; at other times I knew that these addictions were my most profound sources of despair and doom.

When I look back, I loved the secret of it all. The hiding, the lying, the subversive behavior. It made me feel important, it gave me the illusion of freedom, and it felt like I had control. The salacious paradox: I truly felt as though I was more free by having my secrets. The truth: I was a slave to all of it. At the time, it was a fun game for me; I felt useful, busy, and real when I got to play it. I'll sneak out on my free period, get stoned, clean up, come back, play it cool, and get away with it. When I faltered in a couple public-speaking assignments and fell asleep in classes, a couple dear teachers who cared about me called me out on it, I pulled it together just enough to land me at the university of my dreams.

Within a few days at Cornell, I managed to find a handful of girls who welcomed me into their posse, and I was subconsciously thrilled to see that their secret life was as compelling as mine, except their secrets were all constructed around food.

I began counting. One slice of cheese, four leaves of lettuce, two crackers, one cup of tea. The perfect meal—1,500 calories per day, at the most. My friends were beautiful, perfectly thin, and utterly exotic to me, and I chose to follow and copy every bite they took. By the time I'd reached the end of freshman year, I was getting alarmingly thin, about to spend an entire summer dedicated to losing more weight, and loving every second of the charade. Controlling, lying, sneaking, pretending to be eating more—it was strangely thrilling and scary, and I felt free. My diminishing weight garnered the attention of my employers; attention I subconsciously wanted and subconsciously enjoyed.

By the end of that summer, I realized I was in trouble. I was addicted to the control, and while I was watching myself count pieces of cereal, relishing the feeling of my bones against my clothes, I realized that I'd "earned" the glances of my friends—looks that I mistook for admiration and jealousy.

Finally, I called a friend who had also battled with and overcame anorexia and asked her how she'd done it. She told me she wanted to have kids someday, and she knew that if she kept starving herself arbitrarily, her reproductive system would shut itself down and there'd be no option. That one truth was enough to help me turn the ship and get my act together.

I snapped out of it and reined it in. I started to add back what I loved to eat, and I willed myself to enjoy my food. It took a couple of months to get my weight back, but I did it.

Within one year, my other two beloved addictions—tobacco and marijuana—replaced the food control; both would plague me for the ensuing thirty years.

In the early 1990s, after graduating Cornell University with a degree in design, I was taken to a class at Yoga Zone on the Upper East Side, founded by Yogiraj Alan Finger. In my first class, I found the emotional freedom I'd sought in other physical activities. The teacher was kind, supportive, even nurturing. I followed a few teachers there for a few years and realized that I hadn't been breathing properly, nor had I been seeing myself clearly, and I certainly hadn't considered the prospect of loving myself. I caught a real glimpse then, a taste of how true self-love might one day feel—but I was still addicted, with no idea that I shouldn't be.

For those years, I worked in the industry of my dreams—textiles and fashion. First as a woven textile stylist, then an assistant to a gifted designer, then I moved to Northern Italy for just over a year, where I worked for a design firm. I loved my work, meeting heroes like Martin Margiela, traveling, learning a new language, and discovering new boundaries for myself—but I was still struggling to quit substances. I'd roll out my mat almost daily, wherever I was, and do a few postures, listen to my breathing, knowing I needed to shift.

In 1998, sitting at my kitchen table in Turin on a late Sunday afternoon, listening to the sounds of families cooking and talking in the courtyard below, something did shift. I took out a pen and began writing on a paper towel all of the jobs I'd do if I could do anything in the world—and teaching kept landing on the page. Teaching kids, in particular—and I gave notice that I wanted to freelance in New York and went home months later.

During a positively transcendent year of learning and training in Art Education at the New School in New York City, I met Cyndi Lee, who was just about to open OM Yoga on Fourteenth Street. It was a potent time; there were maybe five yoga studios open in the entire city, and we trainees were smitten with her style—her amicability, accountability, openness, and willingness to share her own personal practices deeply benefited us all. From her meditation practices to her style of Hatha vinyasa yoga, we were seeing an original offering, a combination of practices that hadn't quite been taught previously. At the same time, she was committed to learning, and would bring in teachers she respected, studying right alongside us.

Cyndi imprinted upon us the valuable practice of bringing our own flavor and love to our teaching. Our work needn't be relegated to copying a teacher or a style or a body of work. It could be ours, even as we respected the source of the teachings. Cyndi made the yoga personal, and when each of us put that personal offering into practice for ourselves, our classes began resonating with more hearts, more souls. Her personal style made our teachings more universal.

When the training ended, I began teaching at her studio, and I relished that time teaching—I saw myself differently when I was in the seat of the teacher. The struggle disappeared, in its place was a new voice, one that listened prior to speaking. I began the work in earnest then—finding teachers of the Fourth Way, as well as mentors and friends who cared about my well-being. Studying with master teachers for years, learning the best of alignment, anatomy, and architecture. In 2002, I opened my own studio in the SoHo district of New York. With a rent break due to September 11, a big dream to serve, a thirty-thousand dollar loan from a client, and a team of dear friends to stand with me, Virayoga became an international hub for yoga for more than twelve years.

During that time, I eloped, had a son, made myself exceedingly proud, and made a series of questionable choices. I learned, I lived, I loved deeply. I managed to give up substances for more than three years, during a few months prior to conception and until almost two years after the birth of my boy. I watched my mama go through a stem cell transplant for lymphoma and live for another five years. I met gifted life coaches, and I cleared up what had haunted me for decades, which culminated in my getting clean and sober on that fall day in 2014.

The many conversations I'd had with colleagues and teachers like Yogarupa Rod Stryker, Tommy Rosen, and Gabrielle Bernstein made it abundantly clear that my finest work in the world could never be fulfilled if I was high—even infrequently. The hundreds of hours I'd spent practicing yoga, then teaching yoga, along with all the moments staring myself down in a posture or a meditation—I finally realized I was utterly divided within myself and couldn't bring myself together with substances of any kind.

In the summer of 2015, I finished the formal coaching process by writing a letter to each of my parents with the help of my coaches, and read the letters to each of them out loud. These words were meant to absolve them of all the "wrongs" I'd still been inappropriately holding against them, and to apologize for all the ways in which I'd made things unnecessarily personal, alienating and hurting both myself and them. That was a profound healing for us.

Thousands of days engaging in the dance of addiction, I've learned a few things about the indelible impressions of childhood that lead inviolably to the tragic ritual of adulthood doubt. Each time someone in authority diminished me, I *chose* to take it in and make it my truth—and that choice added fuel to the fire of my future addiction. Nobody else had chosen that for me, and nobody can or will be blamed for my circumstances.

So, to the first grade teacher who told me I was too slow, the third grade teacher who told me I was too fast, the fifth grade teacher who made me feel like a criminal for passing a note to a boy I adored—*I forgive the teacher, and I forgive me*. I chose to let you in and make your words part of who I am. And that choice led me to turn on myself time and again, when the option was on the table to run, numb, stop the flow, try to control. Drugs, food, denial, overindulging—it's all the same pain, all the same blaming.

The most salient question for you and me is this: Will we spend the rest of our lives blaming those who put us down and made us feel small, or will we amplify the moment in which we chose otherwise? Will I remember each day from here on out the freedom I found in my own eyes when I reached across time and quit it all, to devise a better way for myself?

Throughout this process, I've learned about my first nature—the path I'd have taken if I hadn't quit—as well as my second nature—the new rituals and restorations that have become the cornerstone of my clarity. Now I'm learning how to make my second nature into my first nature; transforming the most nourishing behaviors into my daily habits. This has taken almost twenty years; it's been a cumulative process, this work of putting intellectual knowing into practical understanding. May you be patient with yourself.

## First Nature

My first nature is a collection of tendencies and practices I'd be able to call mine *if* I'd stayed in my addiction. The daily secrets, hiding, lies, coverup, cleanup, and unkept promises. The pain of wishing and not willing. The volatile temper. The misidentification with substances, food, men. The sadness of knowing there is a better way.

## Second Nature

My second nature is an aggregate of the practices I've undertaken to become who I'm becoming now. Creating beauty through art and music. Empowering myself and others. Generating abundance. Meditating regularly. Trusting myself. Taking time to care for my body, my heart, my mind. Being grateful for my sobriety. Being ready to apologize and to forgive. Cultivating a nurturing circle of friends and family, and keeping them close so I can live true to my highest. Staying in steady communication with my child. Being consistent in my love for my man and holding him closely whenever I can. This is the high I was seeking all that time. The feeling of knowing who I am and knowing where I stand.

I've begun to make these practices my first nature over these past months, with a fair amount of success. One day recently, I found myself sitting at my desk in my home, which is really a beautiful old mirrored coffee table. Light streaming in onto the surface of the table, a brisk cold wind whistled through the long panes of the windows, my collection of crystal singing bowls sparkled on the surface of the table just beyond my laptop, the long arm of my white orchid was reminding me of how to stand elegantly in the sun. It was 1:22 p.m.; I cannot forget that because I had the distinct thought of having arrived in myself, and twenty-two is one of my favorite numbers. It was a sense of quiet knowing, and it was exalted. I smiled to myself. I remember thinking I wanted to call my mom, or someone, to celebrate—but then I thought better of it—since I'd finally learned how to be sober, solo, and steady, I should simply savor this moment on my own. I was free. I was me. I was enough. I had so much. It was almost too much.

Two hours later, I went to pick up my son at school, and he wasn't feeling well. He was meant to accompany me to teach an early evening yoga class in Brooklyn, and he didn't want to; I was scrambling to text a sitter and having no luck, becoming more agitated. I agreed to play his beloved table hockey game in an attempt to bring him around. At 3:45 p.m., I received a frantic phone call. My mom had had a heart attack, and could I stay calm but come straight away.

Two days and one whole lifetime later, Mama had passed. We'd spent that day surrounding her with light, with our voices, with song, with the presence I'd so gratefully noticed just hours before. My sibling and I, over the course of that day she died, became one entity after years of being so separated from one another, and we were both reborn, more purposeful and with intention to carry forward the legacy of our mother's depth of generosity and spirit.

And all I can say, throughout these days, is thank God for my clarity.

My assignments now include staying sober and being a lover. Softness, connectedness, groundedness; the true mother. Engaging in my path publicly has helped me to stay accountable and present to my recovery, and now I have a group of women with whom I'm communicating frequently to help them on their journey. My personal evolution has helped me see that this life is not a problem to be solved but a process of recognition, kindness, and growth. Reliance on a higher power is crucial, belief in my own capacities is crucial, and I have to remember to celebrate simplicity above all.

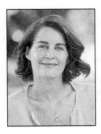

Mama, teacher, speaker, coach, and author, Elena has taught yoga and meditation since 1999. Influenced by several traditions including Katonah Yoga, ParaYoga, and Kundalini Yoga, Elena offers practice as a way to approach our world with realistic reverence and gratitude. Her first book, *x*, has been ranked number one for design on Amazon, and has been translated into five languages. She's an executive producer for *On Meditation*, and founder of Teach.yoga, a virtual home for thousands of yoga teachers worldwide.

Author photo by Sidney Bensimon.

# REBIRTH & RECONNECTION: MY JOURNEY WITH CANCER

## *Dana Byerlee*

This is the hardest thing I've ever had to write. So it's exactly what I must write.

In 2015, I was thirty-four years old. I completed six rounds of chemotherapy for breast cancer, had a mastectomy in which my left breast was removed, and underwent a couple months of radiation.

The year 2015 was also the best year of my life. I know. Inconceivable, but true.

For me, cancer has been a catalyst for rebirth and reconnection to the deepest, most sacred parts of life. It's demolished so many of the paradigms, archetypes, and cultural expectations I unwittingly bought in and forever broke open my heart, which for years had been so closed.

The backbone of all this has been yoga. My yoga practice and, most importantly, the incredible friends I've met from the yoga community gave me the tools and love to not only cope physically and emotionally but also cross that bridge to letting cancer become a spiritual experience. Because it is. Everything is. Triangle pose, washing the dishes pose, having an IV put in you pose ... Whatever you're doing, we can let this practice of life continuously change us, break us, and remold us anew.

## Planting Seeds for the Future

Yoga came into my life when I moved from New York City to Santa Monica. My boyfriend at the time suggested we try it, and I rolled my eyes. *Typical California hippie stuff*, I thought. But I was curious and we went to Travis Eliot's Power Yoga class prepared to do some easy stretching. Needless to say, I got humbled very quickly. It became quite clear I hadn't touched some key muscles since I was a kid, and worst of all, I left confused and angry. I had spent the whole class looking around the room, comparing myself to what other people were doing, and beating myself up for not being stronger or more flexible. But something Travis had said really stuck with me: How can we handle the big challenges of life if we can't stand on our yoga mat without freaking out?

And so I came back.

For years I came to yoga on and off, never practicing consistently. I'd abandon it for months, once even a year, but something always kept pulling me back. I had to admit, there seemed to be a correlation between my time on the mat and the quality of both my inner and outer life. Then one day, somewhat spontaneously, I signed up for Travis and Lauren Eckstrom's 200-hour teacher training. I had no idea that this would be one of the most important and best decisions of my life.

We opened teacher training with a circle to get to know each other, and immediately I felt that these were the kind of people I wanted, needed, in my life. Travis and Lauren said over the next few months we would come to find that yoga is more than just asana, that it's a whole system for living a holistically healthy life, and that some of these new faces in the room would become our lifelong friends. And that's exactly what happened.

I started to become in touch with and aware of my body in ways I never knew possible. After a lifetime suffering with anxiety, I learned how to breathe and better self-regulate. And my heart and mind started to open, as we had some of the most incredible discussions and shared our experiences.

Teacher training finished in June. And then one soul-wrenching meeting in a doctor's office that September, and I was off getting second opinions, weighing my options, and entering a world I never wanted to know. I was told it would be over a year before I was done with all the treatments and surgery. It seemed insurmountable.

Yet in the midst of the terror, I also heard a wisdom telling me if I listened, if I let myself feel the totality of this experience, this could be the most profound experience of my life. I also had a knowing that I had everything I needed, and I understood the miraculous timing of this all. Just a few months before, I had been drawn to that teacher training, at that time and with that particular group of people for a reason. I had been shown the tools to ground through challenging situations, to see beyond the face value of things, and had practiced being physically uncomfortable.

I thought, *Okay, so this will be the ultimate practice. A year-long master class. This is the time to level up and take this yoga practice off the mat.* I decided I would show up to this cancer experience as best I could because, why not? This is it. This is my life, right here, right now, and I don't want to miss another moment more of it.

## Life in the Slow Lane

I hate chair pose, especially twisting chair pose. I have to get so focused when I practice this, mindfully surrender and become immersed in my breath, and remind myself it's just temporary. In a few moments, chair will be over, life will go on.

Naively, I had thought I'd be able to keep working during treatment. Heck, I even thought I'd still be able to go on a yoga retreat to Peru for New Year's! But after that first round of treatment it became clear that for me, the sickness of chemo was like being in twisting chair … twenty-four hours a day, for an entire week. And you can't come out of it to take a break. Chemo pose ends when it says it ends, and you can either fight it (which believe me I tried) or learn to surrender into its dark, time-warped place, letting the chemicals do their job. And just like that, I was on disability. Just the word: Disability. Disabled. Me? I had just been doing push-ups in *chaturanga* the week before. My whole life I'd been neurotically obsessed with achieving, perfecting, pushing, and being busy ... and now my only job was to simply be.

I'd had a daily meditation practice since teacher training, usually ten minutes or so, but now I spent day in and day out tuning in and going deep. I explored loving-kindness, chakra alignment, zazen, and mantra-based meditations, but I especially fell in love with *yoga nidra*, or "yogic sleep" induced by breath and body-scanning. I was amazed at what a powerful game-changer meditation is, and, for me, it totally blew asana away. This was something I could do anywhere, anytime, and it helped me learn to approach confronting moments with more curiosity, objectivity, and mindfulness.

By slowing down, I felt the world come alive again. I was able to see miracles that had always been right under my nose. A cup of sorbet tasted so incredible it blew my mind and brought tears to my eyes. Such a simple thing, not necessary but so delightful, and I understood the real meaning of luxury and was overwhelmed with gratitude. I'd go out after some rare SoCal rain and stand in the middle of the sidewalk, taking in the smell of wet leaves and grass, and cry with amazement. Between treatments I'd set my alarm early, just so I could wake up and lie in bed to take in the incredible luxury of not feeling sick, soaking up that early morning cozy.

Where had I been all these years? It's like I was a kid again, and had suddenly woken up from a twenty-year slumber. Even during these hard times, I felt like the luckiest person in the world.

## Only What Remains Is True

During 2015, everything I associated with my identity was stripped away. Not only was I unable to work, but I also ended a ten-year relationship right in the middle of treatment. And for the first time, I felt terrifyingly uncomfortable in my own skin. I had always been pretty happy with my physical appearance. Maybe even a little vain. Naturally thin and toned, with long thick hair that always got compliments, I'd look at myself in the mirror clothed or naked and think, *Wow, I really lucked out.* I garnered a great deal of confidence, self-worth, and security knowing I met society's expectations of what a woman should look like.

But quickly after treatment that all changed. My appetite was affected and I went from thin to skinny. Though I used something called "Cold Caps" to keep some of my hair, I still had to watch it come out in clumps each day, until it became super thin. I dreaded going out in public and would spend hours crying before leaving. Even at home I wasn't comfortable. I didn't want to see myself in the mirror, and I couldn't shower or dress with the lights on. I didn't want to see my breasts, and I soon became afraid to even touch them.

Asking for help was the scariest and most humbling thing in the world. No longer could I put on my fake Wonder Woman mask and pretend to be okay. After much resistance, my dear friend from teacher training and fellow survivor persuaded me to let people sign up for giving rides, bringing meals, and just checking in and spending time. Letting others into these tender and vulnerable moments was absolutely incredible, and my yoga crew rallied and showed me a depth of love and caring I didn't even know was possible. I was so used to relying on the long-standing social-currency I usually offered—my resume, looks, being someone's girlfriend. But these people didn't care. They didn't care that I had no job or title or moved slowly or what I looked like. They seemed to be happy just spending time with *me*. They were somehow able to see me beyond these messy circumstances. I was shocked. For the first time in my life, I started to think maybe, just maybe, who I am as a person is enough.

## Soul Remembrance

I was so excited when chemo was over and will never forget the night I found out that the latest MRI showed the cancer was gone, fully resolved. But my joy was short-lived. One of the worst days of my life was the day I sat in a room with my whole team of doctors and they told me that they could not save my breast where the tumor had been. Too much of the tissue had been affected and I would have to have an implant. I was beyond devastated. What would it feel like? What would people think? How could I ever be intimate with a guy again? I had thought all these body issues would be a temporary thing, that soon everything would be back to normal.

I spent a week in a dark, dark place and cried bitterly when I heard women on the street talking about plastic surgery as they walked by with their beautiful, healthy breasts. It took all my control to not turn around, pin them against the wall, and scream, "Do you know how lucky you are? I'd give anything to have what you do right now. Who told you your healthy body isn't good enough?" But I knew. The same marketing I'd heard since I was a kid that a woman's value and beauty is based on her appearance. The same voice that had whispered to me at the start of all this that without a good job title or a strong body able to do headstands that no one would want to hang out with me. And finally I truly saw through this bullshit once and for all.

After my surgery, a friend said something I'll never forget: "Dana, implant or not, there's nothing you could ever do to *not* be a woman. Everything about you exudes the feminine. That's your innate energy, and nothing can change that." And that day I looked around my support group of women, many with double mastectomies and still-short, growing hair. There was absolutely nothing unfeminine about them. In fact, they radiated *shakti*, that strong, divine female energy, in a way I hadn't truly noticed before. I realized a woman or man isn't defined by their form. It's their essence.

I had a sudden deeper understanding for the far too many people who are marginalized every day. Whether it's for looks, race, income level, physical ability, sexuality, or age, so many of our fellow women and men are told that they don't deserve to be seen and are treated like ghosts. But who we are is beyond any form we could ever take. Our bodies are simply our vessels to move about in this world. Who we are is that *prana*, that life-force energy, flowing through us. Who we are cannot be seen with the eyes. And incredibly, now with one fake breast, I started to feel *more* feminine than I ever had, and my heart burst open even more with compassion and love.

## Rest Is the New Hustle

As I was both forced and consciously moved to take the pressure off myself, one of the things that changed was my physical asana practice. Before cancer, I usually stuck to power yoga, generally muscling my way through class. I wanted to nail every pose and refused myself breaks. But when I was tired from treatment and rebuilding mobility after surgery, I learned to show myself more compassion. I said to myself one day, "Well, now you have an excuse to skip vinyasas, or go into child's pose whenever you want." Yikes. That had always been an option! But with this new permission, asana really took a leap from just a workout to a healing practice. I listened to my body. I moved to open and heal and strengthen—not to prove something. I was so grateful to be on my mat doing anything and began to think of each movement, even something as simple as a forward bend, as a prayer. I fell madly in love with the sweetness of gentle flows and the magic of restorative yoga. Breath by breath, these practices combined with meditation slowly but surely helped me come back into my body, break down the fear of seeing my post-surgery self in the mirror, and of touching my chest.

My practice has never been the same since. Even today, on the other side of all this, my practice is much more balanced, and so much more personalized. I still do power yoga, but I don't hurry or force. I breathe and move more slowly. I challenge myself when my body, not my mind or ego, encourages me to. And dammit, I take breaks. But now the majority of my practice is gentle, yin, and restorative. Personally, I think I am not alone in my changing practice. The fitness world tends to push high-intensity, yang energy activities like Box-n-Burn, Soul Cycle, and Power Yoga. I love all these things. But people's bodies and minds need balance. All the great athletes know we need time to quiet, repair, and rebuild. In Los Angeles, I notice an increasing interest in gentle, yin, and restorative yoga, as well as meditation and sound baths, and I fully expect this trend to continue and expand.

## Embracing the Paradox

I have a whole list of "Best Cancer Moments." It's pages long now, and includes things from my dad gently washing what was left of my hair in the sink, to the miracle of letting that sweet sorbet melt in my mouth. I think the most important thing I've learned is that nothing is black or white, horrible or good. Contained in every moment, even the most heartbreaking and frightening, there lives a whole paradoxical kaleidoscope of every emotion and feeling, vast and expansive with a vibrant sweetness at the core.

So, 2015 was awful. And magical. And awe-inspiring. But mostly full of so much love. A kind of love for which there is no language, that can feel too much for a human to hold, and that I now know pulses through and unites everything. Everything, person, interaction can become our *upaguru*—Sanskrit for "the teacher right beside you." So don't look away. Don't avert your eyes. We weren't meant to stay trapped in a binary frost of black and white. Only by opening ourselves up to all of life, including the messy, scary, frightening, and heartbreaking, can we finally breathe in technicolor.

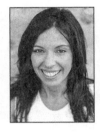

Dana Byerlee is a writer, yoga and meditation teacher, and cancer survivor based in Los Angeles. Yoga has been key to her journey of healing, reclaiming her body, and deep spiritual growth. Dana is passionate about lifestyle and preventative medicine and believes that together the world-wide yoga community can affect radical, positive change. Visit her at www.danabyerlee.com.

Author photo by Rachael Thompson Photography.

# DRAGONS AND OTHER DEMONS

## *Jodi Strock*

"What would you do if you walked into a castle and suddenly a dragon popped out and wanted to eat you?"

I was in first grade, pausing from a game of tag on the playground. Some classmates and I were eagerly discussing this very question. Some kids said they would run. I remember thinking that was pointless. Why would I want to anger him by running away? A big dragon would easily catch me, blow fire on me, and burn me. Other kids said they would fight and kill the dragon. I thought that this was grandiose. How could a small child kill a big, fiery dragon? I distinctly remember thinking I would help the dragon find other food. I would talk to him. I would become his friend so that he would not want to eat me.

## In the Dragon's Den

It was Christmas break and some girlfriends and I went to a dive bar. I was the sober driver that night. Not only was I underage but I was the only one too afraid to attempt using a fake ID. As we entered the dive, I spotted my dragon; only I did not know it. He was incredibly tall, strong, and attractive. My friends and I joked about who would have the courage to approach him. I was just young enough to confuse an ego challenge with confidence. So, I gathered up my sass and walked right over to him.

He was friendly and invited me and my girlfriends back to his dorm room.

We arrived at his small, one-person dorm. I had to use the bathroom and, because it was down the hall, he insisted on walking me to it. I was flattered. He seemed to want to steal a moment alone with me, though I felt some alarm when I had to ask him to leave the bathroom to give me privacy.

As I emerged from the bathroom, I felt a twinge of uncertainty when he suddenly kissed me. Then I thought, *Wow, a really attractive guy is kissing me. This can't be so bad.* Another red flag went up when he started moving me back toward the bathroom door with the pressure of his body against mine. He gently pushed the bathroom door back open and guided our kissing bodies through it.

I'm not sure what prompted me, but I stopped him to tell him that I would not have sex with him. He said "okay" and kept kissing me. Something didn't seem quite right. All at once, he pinned my hands behind my back and hoisted my body onto the counter. The next thing I remember was watching my body get raped, almost like a ghost floating in the upper right hand corner of the bathroom.

Floating above the body is a commonly reported trauma response. It is called disassociating and is a form of the freeze response we undergo as mammals when fight or flight are not a viable option. As a licensed professional and as a result of my own therapy for years, I now have a better understanding of the various responses my body and mind underwent that night. I now understand that those kids on the playground who said they would either run from or fight against the dragon were responding with their fight or flight response. Never did it occur to our innocent, young minds that we could be so ridden with terror that our body would instinctually freeze and our minds would wisely remove our consciousness from the situation. A true testament to how incredible our bodies and minds are.

When he finished with me, I looked at him and whispered, "But I said no." His response terrified me to the core. He said that if I told anyone that this was rape, he would find me and my family and kill us. In an instant of panic I reassured him that I wouldn't tell anyone. I think I even told him I enjoyed it. I went on to ask him all about his family, his past relationships, and childhood. We spent about thirty minutes in the bathroom with him telling me all about how his last girlfriend broke his heart.

As he went on about the intimate details of his family and past relationships, I felt my fear wane. I started to breathe again. I started to feel safe. "The dragon isn't going to kill me if I am his friend."

Dr. Shelley E. Taylor developed the "tend and befriend" theoretical model resulting from her research at UCLA.[1] She found that some animals, primarily female, engage in this behavior as a response to threat. When I first read about this theory, it was a good ten years after I had been raped. However, I immediately felt a sense of ease and relief. It was the first time I was able to understand and release some of the guilt I felt about being so nice to my rapist, moments after he violated me. As a clinician, I have seen this same pattern played out in various stories told to me by clients who have endured rape and other traumas.

Before I came to this understanding I was stuck with this very scary, life-changing thing that happened to me. As an athlete, head of my university's group fitness department, and a sports medicine major, it's no surprise that I turned to exercise to cope. Running myself to exhaustion, lifting weights and then teaching group exercise classes, followed by playing basketball seemed to be the only way I could escape the anxiety, fear, guilt, and anger I was holding deep in my body.

It started as a desire to become stronger and faster in hopes I could keep myself safe. However, exercise quickly became an ample excuse to isolate myself from my friends. If I had to get up early to run or teach an aerobics class, nobody really questioned why I didn't want to go out to parties and bars anymore. The truth was that every time I went to a frat party or out to a bar I became overwhelmed with anxiety. I looked

1. Shelley E. Taylor, Laura Cousino Klein, Brian P. Lewis, Tara L. Gruenewald, Regan A. R. Gurung, and John A. Updegraff, "Biobehavioral Responses to Stress in Females: Tend-and-Befriend, Not Fight-or-Flight," *Psychological Review*, vol. 107, no. 3 (2000): 411–429.

at every single man as a potential threat. Finding joy became impossible. Exercise was one of the only ways I knew how to release this tension. This, mixed with a long history of an eating disorder, body image issues, and struggles with my self-confidence became life-threatening. In my new identity as a personal trainer, fitness instructor, and top student, it became easy to block out that the rape even happened. I remember even thinking, *Wow! I'm really doing an amazing job of not going into my old eating disorder patterns. I must be handling this rape well.* I soon realized, however, that what seemed like a healthier coping skill on the surface was, in fact, exercise bulimia.

I sought "perfection" my entire life. I wanted to be seen as a "fun" girl, while still being able to surprise and delight people with my intelligence and top grades. I wanted to be thin but be seen drinking beer and eating whatever I wanted. I wanted people to see me as a joyful person but know there is a depth to me that could awe them. And, in my mind, all of this came down to what I looked like. I felt so very empty all the time and it seemed that whatever people wanted me to be is what I would fill myself up with for that moment, as an attempt to become their vision of perfection. Thin was the baseline measure of this "perfect girl" I had constructed in my mind thanks to a variety of influences.

When I was six years old, I heard a grown-up say that "metabolism" was something that equated with how much food one could or *should* eat. In my case, I was told I shouldn't eat as many Oreos as my brother because his was faster than mine. From that day until rehab sixteen years later, I stopped eating Oreos. But Oreos were just the beginning of a long line of foods that fell into the "do not eat" category.

And then, one day in high school I collapsed. When my parents took me to the hospital, they put IVs in my arm to give my body the nourishment it desperately needed. I remember being so angry inside! *They are undoing all of my hard work,* I thought. However angry I felt on the inside, I smiled politely and left the hospital. The next days I brutally punished myself through restriction in an attempt to get back to the place I was before they "undid" all my hard work with those IVs.

I do not know how the rape would have impacted me if all of my negative and dysfunctional body image issues had not processed it. Feeling connected to my body was a foreign concept from a very young age. Being raped simply deepened the groove that was already set in place. People often ask how anyone can starve themselves. For me, I was so disconnected from my body that I simply didn't notice anymore. When discomfort would arise, I would restrict a little more, smile a little harder, and try my best to be a "good girl."

## The Many Paths to Healing

I now know, as a licensed marriage and family therapist and rape and eating disorder survivor, that trauma and recovery have their own timeline when it comes to processing and healing. Just because I went to therapy and wanted to deal with the issues right away didn't mean that was the way it happened.

It would be nice to say that I went to a yoga class and all of a sudden the sky opened up and everything turned out wonderful. That is not how it happened for me. And, I don't really believe that is the way it happens for most of us.

Here is what did happen…

About two months after I was raped, a girl from one of my sports medicine classes approached me and told me she was a yoga instructor. She was interested in teaching yoga for our campus fitness department. Since I was in charge of the department, she asked if she could audition for me. This was my first experience with yoga. It was quite a difference from my usual high-intensity experience that took place in that aerobics room. Part of me absolutely hated it. It felt unbearable to be in my body. I couldn't wait for the end. Time seemed to be moving so slow in comparison to my racing mind. I must have looked at the clock 100 times in that hour. Yet, as she guided me into *savasana,* I found a place of peace that I had not experienced since I was a little girl when my mom tucked me into bed. I walked away from that class confused. I hired her and began a semi-regular practice.

A year after I graduated college, approximately three years after my first yoga class, I checked myself into rehab for my eating disorder. It was here that I started gaining a deeper understanding of the trauma I endured from the rape. I also started to look more honestly at my dependency on the approval of everyone outside of myself.

At the inpatient program, I was put on exercise restriction for the first two weeks. The very first day of no exercise I remember sitting on a bench in the common area feeling more discomfort than I had ever felt in my life. I felt as if my muscles were frozen sticks of butter slowly melting away in the heat of the fear in my body. I was so uncomfortable.

Over time, I gained weight, trust, and the privilege to move my body again. The upside of wanting to be seen as perfect is that it provided quite a double bind between my eating disorder's desire to be thin at all costs and my ego's desire to have the staff at the rehab think I was the "best patient ever." Ego worked in my favor here. I started to redefine my definition of desirable. Desirable had now come to mean being more balanced and nourishing my body. While this definition was based on the standards of the treatment center, it was the beginning of what I slowly internalized over the years.

As exercise restriction was lifted, I took the movement class that the rehab offered. The class was a dance and yoga class. This was the first time I experienced yoga as empowering. It felt good to have a space where I could take care of myself and exercise in a way that was gentle and nurturing (instead of a way to manipulate my appearance).

When I got released from the treatment center, I went back to South Carolina, where I had moved after college, and started exploring yoga studios in the area. To my surprise, the type of yoga I found was full of sweaty people (and different from the yoga I was allowed to practice in treatment). The closest studio to my house was an Ashtanga studio. The compulsive exerciser in me was ecstatic to find something that was called yoga and could physically exhaust me. It felt safe and I felt strong.

I did feel a twinge of concern. *What if such a high intensity class could become a new way for me to engage in my old, addictive patterns?* However, I decided not to worry too much about the conflicting views in my mind and started showing up regularly to class. The idea of finding a discipline that allowed me to tune into my body both terrified and appealed to me.

In the months that followed, I noticed that I was starting to cultivate an interest in caring for my body. This was a concept that had previously been so foreign to me. Further, I was beginning to have faith that if I could continue to care for myself I had a lot to offer others.

A year later, I moved out to Los Angeles to pursue a master's degree in psychology. I was both overwhelmed and overjoyed to find that there was no shortage of yoga studios. I found a studio that became my home and my community. My love for yoga grew, as did my love for my community. This studio was a safe place where I could quietly battle my inner struggles. Many days (perhaps, most) were still filled with self-judgment, insecurity, and tears in front of the mirror. I wondered if I would ever "get better." When would I love myself, accept what I saw in the mirror, and not be terrified to breathe into my belly? Despite being tormented with a competitive desire to be "the best yogi in class," I was committed to fostering the voice that was growing inside of me that reminded me this is not about competition. This new voice was hardly loud enough to call a whisper, but it was reserving space for the self-acceptance that I did not yet embody.

I continued to show up on my mat. Slowly, I noticed that when asked to lift all ten of my toes or soften my fingertips, I could feel it. I could actually feel my body. I was in my body. And best of all, it was a safe place to be. And for that moment, I enjoyed it. I found that I started to prefer a yoga class over a run. My interest was peaked by a quiet knowing that the greatest challenge was not manipulating my body into any inversion, arm balance, or pretzel pose but to sit with the discomfort. I started to notice my inner experience range from anger that I wasn't stronger to shame that I may have to come out of the pose before others to frustration that I cared about any of that and so on.

I was amazed at how much the mat was a microcosm for life. There were days I would push myself too hard and days I would get injured. I would show up some days tired. Some days, I would show up and surprise myself with the courage I had to try something new. Other days, I would attempt what was easy the day prior, only to find that I was not able to do it this day. It was through these very literal and physical experiences on my mat that I started to practice how I handled such events outside of the yoga studio.

## Befriending the Dragons Within

I got better at being honest with myself. Part of being honest was admitting I was tired. Resting in child's pose stirred a deep discomfort. Yoga gave me a place to practice being with discomfort in a safe way. The combination of watching how my mind would avoid discomfort and the reminder to return to the discomfort with kindness was a practice that my soul desperately needed and devoured. As my ability to be with discomfort increased, my reactivity seemed to decrease. What I could physically do in a yoga class became far less important than how I was able to care for myself.

Through yoga, meditation, and therapy, I gained an understanding that the freezing, disassociating, and tending and befriending I underwent the night I was raped is proof that I can afford to trust my body/mind/self deeply. Let me explain: it is those responses that kept me safe. There is a wisdom and will to survive that reaches beyond our consciousness. I am grateful to that part of my being. This is one of the many ways in which I have come to have a deeper trust and respect for my body and mind. It is as if there is a wise being inside us all that has our best interest in mind and works toward that even when our conscious mind is not aware. I feel a deep peace when I remember that this is always here inside of me.

In recent years, my practice has been cultivating an internal friendliness that allows a turning toward my insecurities, fears, and self-rejection. I spent so long thinking that I had to get over these parts of myself to find peace. However, in truth, the deepest healing began when I welcomed the challenged parts of myself in. I work to tend and befriend the dragons within.

And in doing so, I learn to love my gifts and care for my shadows.

There was no one yoga class, one *dharma* talk, one teacher, one spiritual practice, or therapist that I credit for the love I have for myself today. It was the accumulation of all my experiences—the complete journey. Through rehab and therapy, I first learned to recognize and tolerate discomfort. Through yoga and meditation, I learned to practice tolerance and grow it into sitting with discomfort. Once I learned to sit with discomfort, I learned how to be compassionate and kind to myself when I experience it. And through the process of it all I have come to make peace with my body and love myself, fully and completely.

Compassion, humility, and acceptance is where my practice lies these days. Taking the yogic path in my recovery has helped me love and trust my body, transform my anger, and nurture myself. This has resulted in me being a better mama, partner, friend, sister, daughter, and therapist. I think it is important to say that meditation, therapy, and yoga do not equate to easy life. In fact, there are moments when my newfound awareness has left me sitting with pain and discomfort that is gut-wrenching. In the past, I would nip this discomfort in the bud by obsessively exercising or restricting my food. Yoga and meditation provide a space for me to practice the important art of self-care. While I no longer struggle with an eating disorder and I enjoy being in my body, there are many other life issues I continue to need this practice for. As it turns out, self-care is never a bad idea.

Yoga was the first space and continues to be the space I return to practice all the things I need to in order for this healing, forgiveness, compassion, and deep change to prosper and evolve. As a result, I am able to carry these gifts out into the world every day.

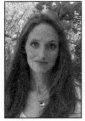

Jodi is a licensed marriage and family therapist working with individuals, couples, and families. She has been trained in the Humanistic Spirituality approach and has a private practice in West Los Angeles. Her background as a family systems therapist incorporates many modalities, including mindfulness, meditation, and inquiry. Her approach combines traditional forms of psychotherapy with Buddhist teachings and yoga practices as well.

Author photo by Justin Strock.

# PART 2 MOVING INWARD & UPWARD

- What have been the most powerful tools or practices on your journey to self-acceptance and wholeness?
- What are you willing to try in order to unapologetically grow into your full authentic self?
- What three things can you commit to today to begin to create peace with yourself?
- Name someone who inspires or supports you on your healing journey.

# PART THREE

## *Yoga for Every Body and Every One*

*Every* body is a "yoga body." In the grassroots movement for inclusion, this has become a common catchphrase, one utilized frequently by the Yoga and Body Image Coalition as well as many other advocates and activists for a body-positive, all-inclusive, and accessible cultural projection and practice of yoga. The writers in this section pose tough questions and invite us to look closely at why yoga remains inaccessible to many and why it's so necessary to continue to reverse this trend and create a new norm.

The epitome of the "yoga body," Gwen Soffer was plagued by a lifetime of whittling away a body that took up too much space. The external rewards were great, encouraging her to continue to exert a tremendous amount of time and energy on maintaining the "ideal" until the veneer cracked and her practice became a place of solace marked by acceptance with no size requirement.

Jacoby Ballard reminds us that self-love is a journey, one that winds and turns and requires vigilance and introspection. Loving ourselves isn't always instantaneous or easy. Our relationships with our selves require effort (like any long-lasting and meaningful relationship). Sharing his own journey, practicing with pain, exposing old wounds and turning toward his whole self, Ballard demonstrates how he has made love a daily practice.

Bullied in elementary school and far removed from the myopic representations of beauty found on TV and in movies, Jessamyn Stanley was saddled with insecurities and a deep sense of self-loathing. Ironically, the seeds of transformation came from two unlikely places— Westernized, studio-culture yoga, often perceived as something only affluent, thin, white women practice, and the bikini + beach saturated world of yoga on social media. Stanley quickly had a practice and a medium to work through and document her journey to self-love, and she offered a new picture of yoga to inspire and validate others en masse.

North America has seen an explosion of yoga in mainstream culture over the last seventeen years, growing out of a fair amount of obscurity to a full-blown cultural phenomenon utilized by corporations to sell products, services, and lifestyle brands. As an Indian American, Lakshmi Nair shares the strange and contradictory space she occupies in conventional yoga spaces. In advocating for accessibility, she encourages us to examine the intersection of consumerism, racism, and cultural appropriation while sharing the need for safe spaces for people of color as a necessity for healing and as a form of social justice.

Sabrina Strings continues with what many may view as an uncomfortable and triggering conversation about the covert racism within yoga culture, a reality that is a reflection of the culture at large. In today's charged political climate, it's a familiar refrain to hear people claim that racism is a thing of the past and that, certainly, it couldn't exist in a "spiritual" place such as in a yoga class. Strings offers evidence to the contrary. She reminds us that if we're committed to making yoga available to everyone, we must also ensure that those yoga spaces are safe and welcoming as well. That end can only be reached if we can begin by listening to the experiences of those who have felt marginalized and excluded.

A lack of representation and a cultural value system that continues to equate female "beauty" as the most worthwhile goal for girls and women resulted in body dysmorphia and disordered eating for Chanelle John.

The rewards of meditation and her burgeoning yoga practice proved to be healing. They inspired her not only to seek out more diverse and accessible yoga spaces but to create them. She reminds us that everyone is valuable and, though it may be challenging, we all benefit from unraveling the structures that oppress us through our collective liberation.

# TAKE UP SPACE AND BE SEEN

## *Gwen Soffer*

How often have we convinced ourselves that we need to be smaller and take up less space? When I was younger, I often thought I was too big: too tall, too heavy, and my feet were even too large. I grew up as a tall girl with an athletic body and curly hair—the trifecta of negative characteristics in my mind. I spent many hours as a young girl and teenager trying to be smaller, which included disordered eating patterns, sneaking diet pills, and pledging to starve myself until I could make this happen. My hair even took up too much space, and I continually struggled to tame my curly locks in the hopes of having perfectly coiffed Dorothy Hamill hair. I would go to bed every night with my hair wet, smooth it down, sleep on one side and then switch midway through the night to attempt to flatten the other side, only to wake up to my uncontrollable ringlets of shame the next morning.

One of the benefits of middle age is that it can be a time of clarity about things that used to be quite overwhelming earlier in life. Sometime around when I turned forty, I had an epiphany about how much time I was wasting trying to get smaller. It occurred to me one day, "What if I did not worry about weight? What if I decided to not buy into the constant preoccupation, not eventually, but right this very minute? Is it possible for me to be present in whatever form my body is in this moment and be ENOUGH?" Amazingly, but not without a lot of work and constant reinforcement, I followed my "WTF!" with a "No more!" Of course, I have flashbacks to old beliefs, but I am committed to inhabiting this body, the one I live in today, with bold and unapologetic compassion. My body no longer was something that I forced to change but instead a vehicle that allowed me to live a full life. With this proclamation, I realized that I already had the tool at my fingertips to help me in this practice of self-acceptance, but I had been misusing it for so many years—yoga.

## Hiding in My "Yoga Body"

When I first discovered yoga, I used it as just another way to perpetuate my destructive belief that my body was not good enough. It provided me secret access to a body that I had been looking for all of my younger life and, by obsessing over it, I was able to find the skinny body that I had been seeking for so long. The results were intoxicating. I got down to a size four, a size that my frame is not meant to hold. When you lose a lot of weight, people start to reinforce the value of being small by telling you how good you look and eagerly asking you how you did it. Of course, there is no malice in these compliments and questions, only other people who have been told "small is better" for a lifetime just like you. I fit the "ideal" of the yoga teacher that we see so often on the cover of yoga magazines and social media, and I remember thinking somehow I had arrived, and I was desperate not to let it go.

This "yoga body" was not without a hefty price, and it took an incredible amount of effort to keep it up. I would wake up at five o'clock every morning to go to a step aerobics class at the gym (warming up for twenty minutes on the rowing machine beforehand), go to a very physical martial arts class at noon, and then squeeze in a yoga class, capping off the day with some sit-ups and push-ups next to my bed before I went to sleep. I was obsessive about what I would and would not eat, and every bite was planned out each and every day. Forcing myself to be small took up a lot of my time and energy, but at the time, it felt worth it, and I justified it in the disguise of health. I finally got what I had wished for—except for the curly hair, I seemed to fit the ideal on the surface. Like any facade, however, it was not sustainable, and eventually the other shoe dropped (still a size 10).

## Practicing Self-Acceptance

The truth is I was using this image to cover up very serious personal issues that I needed to face. For as long as I can remember, I have struggled with depression. I am an upbeat, independent, and productive person, so it was always easy to hide this from people, including myself, but it had gotten much worse. The "yoga body" that I had was actually the result of this hidden depression, and I was self-medicating through disordered eating, alcohol abuse, and obsessive exercise. I fit the portrayed yoga ideal, however, and it went unquestioned. I was able to continue my destructive behavior right out in the open without anyone paying attention, and I could get a quick fix anytime I felt down. The most dangerous part of this avoidance technique was how abusive I had become to my own psyche. Because skinny is equated to being happy, well-adjusted, and confident, it is easy to hide this type of self-destruction. I was in complete denial that underneath the image I was falling apart, and the relationships that meant the most to me were suffering. Instead of spending my time and energy building myself as a person, I was losing who I was at the core. The truth, however, has a way of making its way to the top, and I could not sustain the act any longer.

After a bad accident falling headfirst down a flight of stairs, I had to step out of yoga for a while, and for the first time in years I went to see a doctor. It had been so easy to keep up appearances before, but now as I sat before him bruised, stitched, and broken, reality was coming to the surface. I remember thinking that I was going to die during my plummet down the stairs, and, in some distorted way, it was the literal and figurative bottom I needed to hit in order to change. My physician had a history of depression and alcohol abuse in his family, and he knew how to ask the right questions that would get to the core of the problem hidden deep down behind the "perfect" yoga facade. He traced my behaviors and addressed my issue with depression and alcohol abuse in a compassionate way, and I was finally able to see what was happening to me. I left his office that day and everything looked different.

It has been almost ten years since that day, and I look a lot different now. I stopped drinking completely, I dropped my gym membership, I began managing my depression, I gained thirty pounds, and I have never felt more confident and self-accepting as I do today approaching age fifty. The path to self-acceptance was not about learning to love my body but more about learning to love myself so that I could show up in the world for real. With my realization that I did not want to spend my energy trying to change my body anymore, I instead started focusing on the freedom and potential that self-acceptance would bring me. As a result, my yoga practice changed drastically. I did not want to abuse it anymore and use it to reinforce my old destructive beliefs about myself, but I wanted to use it to establish sustainable self-acceptance that would then push me into the real work that I am here to do.

Yoga became a practice of being with myself no matter what my outer shell looked like and no matter what I was struggling with. It became a practice without judgment that was liberating in a way that I had not experienced before. We are taught from a very young age that we only deserve to feel free in our bodies if we look a certain way. We are taught that if we do not fit the model of beauty that we should be shamed about our body and that we don't deserve to be seen.

After a beginner yoga workshop that I taught recently, I asked the participants to fill out a questionnaire. One of the questions was, "Why have you not tried yoga sooner?" Overwhelmingly, the responses were based on not believing they had a "good enough" body to practice yoga: too heavy, too inflexible, too old, too uncoordinated, not like the images they had seen of yogis. This really struck deep for me, and I understand why they would feel this way. Saying that yoga is for everyone is not enough if our classes and teachers don't reflect everyone. The truth is that many people feel that they don't deserve to be seen if they do not match the ideals that we perpetuate in our media, including the yoga media.

## Taking Up Your Space

With the change in my own yoga practice came a change in how I teach yoga. I started to pay more attention to what I was saying and how I was instructing poses. I began instructing a wider stance in poses, including expansion in the arms, grounding in the hips, and embracing the power of our bodies. I often use the expression, "Take up your space on your mat," and students tell me how powerful it feels when they give themselves permission to get big. How many times have we been told in our lives to get small? Whether it is getting smaller in our bodies, in our voice, in our opinions—there are too many to count—and it feels good to stand tall. In order to do this, we have to be willing to fill our space and be seen.

Being seen is a crucial element in our emotional well-being. When we are babies, we instinctively look to those around us for affirmation of our safety and validation of our worth. You see me. You hear me. You understand me. You care about me. I trust you. I am enough. We are hardwired to look at each other, and our emotional development depends on knowing others value us and that we matter. Being seen goes far deeper than what we project on the outside, but we have been told over and over again that our bodies represent who we are. When we don't take up our space, we are in essence trying not to be seen for fear of rejection, so getting small has become, for many, a way to protect ourselves.

In my women's self-defense classes, I point out to my students that women have their power in their hips, which makes them amazing kickers. I make the connection that the place where women are the strongest, their hips and legs, is exactly where we are often told to get smaller. Not a coincidence. We talk about how to use our strength and not to deny it or struggle to make our power smaller. Helping women see that they are powerful in their minds and hearts and also in their bodies is so important. So many of us have grown up believing that the place of our physical power is not beautiful if it is too big. So, what do we do? We spend hours complaining about this power spot and even more hours working to get rid of it. In yoga terms, our body is our "first home" with the grounding energy of the first chakra in the lower part of the body. This energy center is where we find safety. It strikes me that if we don't believe we are enough in our first home, our bodies, how will we move completely into our own power in our lives?

What I love most about teaching yoga and self-defense is when I see women begin to realize how powerful they actually are. I can see in the way that they stand and the expression in their face that they are intentionally filling their space. It is very liberating to use the power of our hips and legs to ground so that we can expand and lead from the heart. Filling your space is not the same as pretending to be big, which involves posturing to appear larger. We don't need to "act" small or "act" big, but instead we can fill our space completely in the body we have without asking permission to do so.

## Being Seen

As a mother, it has always been important to me to teach my daughter how to take up space, be seen, and not ask permission or apologize for it. Although I struggled when she was younger to negotiate the constant cultural and media images that pressured her to do otherwise, I was relentless in pointing out the false ideal that she was seeing. More importantly, I knew I had to live by example by taking up my space unapologetically. I knew that my opinion of myself and my willingness to be seen was the anchor that would bring her back to understanding her own power. I wanted her to know that how she treats herself and others and how she shows up in the world is always more important than appearances. Because of the hundreds of images that our young girls are seeing every day telling them to "be smaller," it is even more important that we take up our space and be seen as mothers, mentors, and teachers—our children are watching us too.

Not always an easy task since we have grown up with the same bombardment of images and finding that confidence can be a real challenge. Yoga for me is now a practice of being myself so that I can step off of my mat and be seen in my world. This practice has helped me negotiate the many conflicts I have had around depression, alcohol abuse, disordered eating, and obsessive exercising, and it has become a safe place that I get to practice a healthier, stronger, and more sustainable relationship with myself. I had to face what exactly I was practicing on my mat, and yoga became the tool that showed me how to deconstruct my belief system so that I could reorder things and start living as the larger, more authentic version of myself. Even if we are not feeling particularly powerful in our lives, we have the space on our mat that is ours to see what it feels like to take up our space. If we practice taking up space, feeling the power of our hips, the openness of our hearts, and our ability to get big, we may just start to understand how much we can fill up our own lives and demand to be seen.

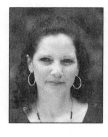

Gwen Soffer is a trauma-informed yoga teacher, women's self-defense instructor, author, and community mentor. She is cofounder of Enso studio in Media, Pennsylvania, and leads trauma-sensitive yoga classes for survivors of trauma. She believes in the strength of the human spirit and is committed to creating safe and empowering spaces for her students to heal. Visit her at www.experienceenso.com.

Author photo by Andy Shelter.

# LEARNING TO LOVE THE WHOLE

## *Jacoby Ballard*

My journey of self-love begins with two invitations that pointed me toward old wounds and, ultimately, healing.

## Invitation #1

"Who hurt you?" was the question that my teacher asked as I approached her through the chanting and candles of the sacred ceremony for my 200-hour yoga teacher training graduation. I didn't know how to answer her, for I saw others be hurt and in their healing process, but I didn't think of myself that way. The only thing that I could think of, that I was in relationship to at the time, was my dad's death when I was six, but that didn't feel like an answer to the question my teacher was asking. Perhaps because I was raised by an independent single mom, strong and resilient, who just kept on keeping on, regardless of what pain happened in our lives. Or perhaps it was due to my own study and practice of social justice, for as I became aware of my white privilege in the world, how could I possibly allow for my own pain to be valid amongst what seemed like the greater pain of people of color, undocumented immigrants, and incarcerated people. In that moment, I told Jaya Devi, "I don't know," but I hung on to the question, it felt like a very important inquiry in my own process of *svadhyaya*, or self-study. She was inviting me, ushering me, toward my pain—both pain that I had sequestered for years and pain that was just around the bend for me.

## Invitation #2

"Now we are going to offer gratitude for the body … thank you, body. Thank you for all that you allow me to experience: the positive, negative, and neutral. Thank you. Thank you, hair follicles, for the warmth and character you create, thank you. Thank you, eyebrows, for keeping the dust out of my eyes, thank you … " I went to a meditation at a retreat for our worker-owned cooperative, this was how we were starting the day, and I was crying as I sat amongst my colleagues, who were mixed race, disabled, black, Latina, fat, gay, white, able-bodied, straight, trans, in their twenties, in their sixties. This felt like the perfect place to grieve and investigate this pain that my tears were evidence of. I had been hating my body, in various ways, since I was an adolescent, and yet I had already been teaching yoga for a decade—a teaching that includes listening to, appreciating, and coming to understand one's body. I had studied the impact of media messages of the "perfect body" and politically critiqued it and validated the many other shapes of bodies, but it felt like quite a different thing to offer my own imperfect, healing body love and gratitude.

## Not Quite Love

Of course, there are many times when I appreciated my body's power— in hiking up 14,000-foot mountains in my home state of Colorado, on the soccer field or basketball court, in orgasm, in witnessing the healing process from injuries and sickness. As an athlete, I wasn't completely disconnected. I learned that my body was something that I could force to do amazing feats—to run ten "suicides" in basketball practice; to bike and hike over mountain passes and peaks, a 5,000-foot elevation gain and many miles; to sprint up hills, from telephone wire post to the next post in soccer practice, training to be able to outrun any other team. I learned a sense of empowerment and awe of my body, but not gratitude, not love.

I honor the way that my own process with my body—the dissociation, self-hatred, the way I hid—got me through difficult times, for as I learn about trauma, I see that each was a coping mechanism that I employed in order to survive. I learned to detach from my body at an early age, at seven when I was sexually abused. I learned that if my mind and attention went elsewhere, I could make it through whatever was happening to my body, rejoin my body later, and move on. In high school, when I faced daily bullying and every day was a trial, I learned that if I could control my eating and therefore my body size, and have something closer to the "ideal" for a young woman, then I could mitigate some of the cruelty directed at me. When I came out as genderqueer and began binding my breasts tightly, beginning with ace bandages and then binding "shirts" with Velcro, hiding my breasts meant I was less often identified as a "woman." If I could be seen as more androgynous, which was who I was on the inside, I felt sexy, handsome, and invincible.

Each of these techniques was a valiant effort at survival. They got me through immense pain that I was not equipped to address. And each of these techniques produced harm for myself in the long-term, preventing me from being fully present in the moment, avoiding conflict, and harming my body. What was intended as a short-term intervention became a long-term unconscious pattern that I have had to consciously unlearn.

## Practicing with Pain

At age seventeen, I began meditating as part of a senior project at my high school. I didn't know anyone who meditated nor read any books or articles about it, but somehow it had seeped into my consciousness. During my senior year, my meditation practice improved my free-throw shot to nearly perfect, cementing my commitment to my sitting practice. At age nineteen, I began an embodied yoga practice as part of a "wellness credit" at my college, taught by a seventy-year-old woman whose photograph remains on my altar to this day, whose life had been completely transformed by the practice. Meditation, asana, and the philosophies of Buddhism and yoga have again and again been healing, directing me toward my shadows, pain, and humanity, and ultimately to love and grace. I have come out as trans through my practice. I have come out as a survivor of childhood sexual abuse through my practice, grieved my grandmother's death through my practice, and faced breakups in a small queer community through my practice. My practice has led me to forgive my foes and to ask for forgiveness from my ex-partner and my mother. My practice has given me the tools to stay present with the pain of the world, from surveillance of Muslim communities to police brutality against black people to the weekly, sometimes daily, homicide of transpeople, often transwomen of color, to the reality of climate change and environmental destruction, and to offer compassion out of mindfulness.

Dissociating from my body became a habit long after high school that would surface not just at moments when I was genuinely threatened but at times when I needed to be the most present in my body and when conditions were "safe." My body could not distinguish between safety and danger, and even in the most loving of sexual acts, my mind and attention would travel elsewhere. Conversely, with sexual partners that I was not sure about, I would also dissociate and come back to the moment either during something that I did not actually want to do or afterward, which would produce incredible shame and grief. Whereas if I had remained present, perhaps I could have stopped something that I did not want from happening. I would dissociate in yoga class, and then find myself in a deeper backbend than was safe for me emotionally and physically. I would dissociate on the phone with my mother, during justice rallies and marches, and during dinner with friends. As my yoga practice evolved, I became increasingly aware of this pattern and I would watch it happen, almost like watching a movie.

In my advanced teacher training, during a meditation module, I efforted to stay in my body during one particular day of meditation, two days into Noble Silence. In the early afternoon, as I attended to sensations in my low abdomen, memories of my childhood sexual abuse surfaced, something I had buried for twenty years. I was flooded with tears for the remainder of the day as my body remembered. I stayed present to the sensations of hot tears dripping onto my cheeks, and I used my practice to feel my sit bones on my cushion and my shins on the ground. I knew that I needed to stay with the sensations and the memories associated with those sensations, that staying may lead to healing.

## Can I Create Less Harm in This Moment?

In high school, my eating disorder was an effort to control something that was beyond my control: bullying. If I could look cute enough, I imagined that I could have a boyfriend, which would stop my peers in their tracks, for they taunted me and gossiped about me, girls would not change next to me in the locker room, and I had few friends, for being gay. I didn't really want a boyfriend, I just wanted the endless shaming, blaming, and surveillance to stop. So, I began to hate my belly, specifically, and control my eating and body weight. And it wasn't until that gratitude meditation with my friend and colleague, that I realized the constant and unconscious harm that I was inflicting.

During a high school soccer practice, one of my teammates had approached me at a break, saying, "Jacoby, why are you doing this?" I had just fallen over from being tackled, but she said that my teammate barely brushed me. I tried to play dumb, but I knew that she saw my pain and vulnerability. I also did not trust her—she was alternately a bystander and a participant in the bullying. Her words did jolt me, not enough to stop but enough to hide my disorder better. This pattern continued into college until a friend told me that she could not be my therapist, and she encouraged me to seek one at the campus health center. Out of a stroke of luck or a godsend, the therapist to whom I was assigned was a woman of color and a justice activist. She connected my eating disorder to my need for control, and she showed me how to examine that pattern in my relationships and activism. She encouraged my yoga and meditation practice, serving to connect my own harmful patterns in my life to the transformation that inevitably occurs on the cushion and mat.

During a visit to New York City at age twenty-four that would lead me to move there a year later, a good friend gave me his old binder. I remember thinking, *Am I really going to do this? Is this really who I am?* as if donning the binder required both courage and commitment. For the next several years, I wore it anytime I was not in my bedroom. When

I practiced yoga in my room, I didn't wear it, testing out whether my aversion to my breasts was others seeing them or me having them. When I practiced in yoga classes, I wore my binder, testing out how I could move, breathe, and be seen as a genderqueer and trans person. As a yogi, I felt my transition into being trans-identified as a spiritual process, and I wanted to move slowly. In New York City, wearing a binder was a commitment in the summertime, for the sun scorched above and the asphalt radiated that heat up from below. Having something compressing my torso and a fabric not quite breathable meant months of being continuously sweaty, my skin being irritated, and being in a grumpy, exasperated mood.

A few years later, I spoke to my teacher about my practice and the impact of my binder: I couldn't often take a deep breath, my shoulders were rounding forward, I sometimes experienced tingling down my arms, and chest-openers were impaired. She told me with such compassion, "It's never okay to hurt yourself." Those words helped move me toward top-surgery. I clearly felt more myself with a flat chest and binding was creating long-term harm, so surgery seemed the obvious means to have both a flat chest and do less harm to my body. It was a permanent choice that I made with intention, clarity, and compassion, guided by my teacher's words.

Many trans and gender nonconforming people bind and tuck daily, and those are often the cheapest options to be seen and to feel ourselves for who we are. Some people engage these methods in the short-term, some engage them long-term. Surgeries are expensive, and in order to access them, trans people need a letter from a therapist saying we've been living as our gender and do indeed have "gender identity disorder" (recently updated in the DSM to "gender dysphoria"). Thus, we have to be diagnosed with a mental disorder in order to access the care we need for our well-being and, sometimes, our survival. Both class and the medical industrial complex are gatekeepers to the treatments that we need, our striving for self-determination intersecting with further barriers created racism, ableism, and fatphobia.

I was earning eight dollars per hour working at a natural food store, and did not have anything to fall back on. I did not have insurance, and chest surgery cost $7,500 out-of-pocket at the time. I began saving money, which was difficult in New York City, especially on my wage. I was also fired for being trans during that time that I saved for surgery, adding further trauma and financial obstacles just for being myself and seeking well-being. I held two fund-raisers, one as a house party and one as a cabaret, complete with MC and art auction. I turned toward my community for help, baring my story and aspiration, and they showed up; through the fund-raisers, a send-off party before surgery, and care during and after surgery, my beloved community was there for me, a beautiful manifestation of the Buddhist refuge of *sangha*.

## Love As a Daily Practice

My practice has allowed me to be all of myself, and to let all of myself be seen, without regret, guilt, or shame. My practice, supported by my teachers, mentors, and collaborators, has taught me that in turning toward my whole self, all of my experiences, I can relate to so many others who have either been through similar pain or any kind of dissociating or self-harm or suffering in general. I have learned to notice when my old coping strategies resurface, and, over time, they surface less and less or don't last as long. I greet them as an old friend, and then send them on their way. As I turn toward my own pain, my capacity to bear witness to the pain of the world increases, for I can notice what is triggered or stirred within me, talk through it with friends and collaborators, root into my practices and resources, and respond with kindness, integrity, clarity, and attention. My process is not and will never be perfect, but each moment is an opportunity to practice creating the world that I want to live in, again and again.

Now I know who and what has hurt me, and I try to address that question and forgive the harm week-by-week, not allowing it to be buried but noticing its impact. I offer my body daily kindness and care, moving toward love of even my belly—a belly and a body not portrayed in commercials or magazines as "ideal." But this is the only body that I will ever have and why waste time *not* loving it?

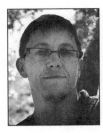

Jacoby Ballard, E-RYT 500, is a white, working-class, genderqueer social justice worker who has been teaching yoga and meditation for seventeen years. He is delighted that within the past five years, his worlds of justice and embodied practice are converging and intersecting in addressing trauma, the pursuit of anti-racism, and shifting our yoga and meditation spaces to explicitly address privilege and oppression.

Author photo by Laurel Schultheis.

# INSTAGRAM, YOGA, AND LEARNING TO LOVE MY BIG, BLACK BODY

## Jessamyn Stanley

White beauty ideals invaded my psyche at a very young age. I'm sure every little black girl has a story just like mine, but please indulge me for a moment. I was encouraged to idolize women who looked absolutely nothing like me. Was it Jennifer Love Hewitt's giant ivory breasts and tiny waist in *Can't Hardly Wait*? Maybe it was Julia Roberts's flowing auburn locks in *Pretty Woman*. I'm sure Alicia Silverstone's iconic portrayal of *Clueless'* avidly blonde and beautiful Cher Horowitz deserves at least a smidge of responsibility. And lest we forget the age of "innocence" at the turn of the twenty-first century when women like Britney Spears and Christina Aguilera dominated and turned the antiquated beauty and body ideals of Edith Wharton's *Age of Innocence* on its ear. Images of slender human Barbie dolls "shuffle-ball changed" their way across my mind when I was both awake and asleep. I prayed every night that I'd wake up with pore-less skin, silky flowing hair, and large, clear azure eyes. I figured I could purchase at least a few of these qualities via, at the very least, consistent investments in Biore pore strips, kanekalon hair extensions, and colored contact lenses. Instead, I woke up every day with acne prone skin, brutally kinky hair, and squinty, almond-ish brown eyes. Because I failed to spontaneously transform into the celebrated beauty icons of the late twentieth century, I considered myself a human failure and thus began a slippery slope toward self-loathing.

When you are hell-bent on a path of vicious self-loathing, a self-fulfilling prophecy is basically wholly ensured. To that end, my adolescence was rough. I was considered heavier, effortlessly awkward, and hadn't quite figured out how to control my body odor and skin dryness. My hair was always acting out against me, and even though I wore complicated braided extensions for most of my adolescence, I quickly acquired the unfortunate nickname of "Medusa" because of the fear inspired by my artificially long locks. What started as an elementary school addiction to French fries and chicken nuggets quickly (and literally) ballooned into a body size that neither Limited Too nor Gap Kids could handle. To be frank, they weren't ready for this jelly. In short, I felt indescribably uncomfortable in my own body and, what's worse, I felt completely alone.

## Does It Really Get Better?

I was bullied by my elementary and middle school classmates to the point of spending all of eighth grade applying for scholarships to attend a semi-local all-girls boarding school. Leaving to attend Salem Academy seemed like an opportunity for change, and I envisioned a future with fewer asinine young men marring my daily life with their endless searing taunts. And, with the help of large scholarships and financial aid, I was welcomed into a sisterhood of intelligent, driven women who were essentially required to value themselves outside of beauty norms.

If fat black girls couldn't be found on MTV or VH1, you certainly couldn't find them in *Seventeen* magazine. But let's face it, they weren't in *Jet* magazine or on B.E.T. (Black Entertainment Television) either. Sure, there were some black bodies on display, but even the fattest among them looked more like Naomi Campbell and Halle Berry than Gabourey Sidibe. There were so few black, female, plus-size role models that I was usually shocked to see someone who looked anything like me on screen or in print. Eventually, the entertainment world started to shed more light on veteran performers like Mo'Nique and Queen Latifah, but aside from those grand queens of comedy and hip-hop, there were a precious few fat black women accepted by or represented in Western media.

I think that's how fat black women learned to laugh at our bodies because our only strong role models were forced to make a career out of laughing at theirs. And I did laugh at my body. I laughed my way from dance performances in elementary school to lead roles in my middle and high school theater programs. I quickly learned that if I could make a joke out of my God-given body, I was one step closer to being accepted by my peers. Turning self-loathing into comedy isn't a terrible method of living life. People do it every day and some have built impressive careers revolving around self-deprecation.

However, my penchant for making a joke of my own insecurities hit a serious roadblock after college. It was hard enough to joke about my body insecurities since I was already a Weight Watchers drop-out three times over and had never been able to maintain a regular gym or eating schedule. But with a host of new insecurities on the horizon, including a crumbling long-term relationship with my high school sweetheart, crippling anxiety over my student loan debt and chosen career path, and an increasing familiarity with the death of loved ones, it became impossible to differentiate my self-loathing from reality.

## "But Isn't Yoga Only for Rich White Girls?"

It probably seems improbable that one of the whitest corners of the fitness world would help change my mental body conversation. We can tap dance around the race, body image, and athletic world crossroads forever, but I'd argue that our inability to accept reality is part of a larger problem. Frankly, the Western yoga world has been heavily fortified by wealthy white America for decades. Up until the late twentieth century, it was extremely uncommon to see a yoga practitioner who wasn't either a stern but svelte brown skinned man or an equally stern but svelte white skinned woman. Before the Internet was part of our daily lives, any other body type besides these two was relatively invisible within the yoga community, and the media has reflected that cultural imbalance. It seems that the Achilles heel of Western yoga is our inability to accept that the eight limbed path knows no "ideal" practitioner. Yoga transcends specific body types, and the practice should be enjoyed by any and all who encounter it.

However, I didn't know about any of that when I started regularly attending Bikram yoga classes around the corner from my graduate school about five years ago. My depression must have been palpable to those around me because one of my grad school classmates encouraged me incessantly to join her in hot yoga classes, which had allowed for considerable emotional clarity in her own life. I wasn't unfamiliar with the idea of a curvy yoga practitioner. My mother has always been interested in holistic healing, and the books and magazines she left strewn about my childhood home made me familiar with the work of Dianne Bondy and Anna Guest-Jelly. I knew there were definitely plus-size women who were practicing yoga and loving it, but their influence hadn't completely punctured my psyche. Quite frankly, the journey toward asana varies from person to person. Usually, the motivation that brings a person to a long-standing yoga practice isn't based upon visibility of body types, but on a desire to truly look within and deconstruct the soul.

Ultimately, what brought me into Winston-Salem, North Carolina's Bikram Yoga studio in 2011 was a need to reclaim my dignity from the angrily clenched fists of depression. To dilute that soul reclamation to the influence of a few curvy bodied practitioners would be off base. Ultimately, I just wanted to stop feeling depressed. When I finally dragged my ass into the studio on Fayette Street, I was shocked to find that a sequence of arduous yoga poses combined with brutally intense breathing exercises was the exact medicine I needed to pull myself out of my life funk.

The extreme heat of the yoga studio, topping out around 105 degrees on a regular basis, was the equivalent of a chloroform soaked rag over the mouth of my self-loathing. Regardless of whatever pathetic quantity of self-doubt and pity I'd brought with me into the studio, it was imperative that I release my baggage in order to make it out of class alive. And when I challenged myself to release my self-doubt and avoid self-pity, I was astounded by the strength my body unleashed. The more I devoted myself to my yoga practice, I saw that my real problems didn't have anything to do with my body or my life circumstances. I began to realize that my perspective and judgment was clouded by my inability to harness my own strength. I saw that the energy I spent showering myself with negativity was primarily responsible for my unhappiness. Every time I practiced, with sweat dripping from my knee creases and tears welling in my eyes, I reclaimed a sense of self-respect that had been sorely missing from my daily life. For me, it was finally a way I could exercise my body and keep the pressures of twenty-first–century body norms at bay.

Sure, my local yoga studios were dominated by plenty of svelte bodies, but how was that any different from an afternoon spent exercising at the YMCA? However, unlike spin classes or treadmill jogs, yoga was a way to look inside myself. Prior to establishing a yoga practice, I never challenged myself to look within my own being for answers to life's endless questions. Up until that point, I remained convinced that the answers to every question could be purchased at the right price or learned at the hands of another human being. By looking within myself, I was finally able to redirect my emotional distress into a respectful internal dialogue. Basically, I was able to discover a way to love myself without the involvement of other people.

## Take a Picture, It'll Last Longer

My true journey toward self-love didn't fully kick into gear until I began regularly photographing my home asana practice and posting the evidence on my Instagram account. I began photographing myself because I noticed a growing number of yoga practitioners and teachers posting asana progress photos on Instagram and I wanted to be part of a larger community. In many ways, home yoga practice can be very isolating, and I wanted to feel like I was "part of a team." In many ways, photographing my body's gradual transition in yoga poses became a kind of guerilla emotional therapy. I transformed into my own psychiatrist and gave myself the necessary time and space to confront my internal demons. By photographing my body and being forced to stare at it on a daily basis, I had a literal constant confrontation with the parts of myself that previously seemed unforgivable. For example, if I photograph myself in the heat of a challenging side plank variation and the image is dominated by my gelatinous fat spilling over the waistband of my leggings, I'm faced with two options: throw shade at my body for not being slender, OR give myself a high five because "DAMN, MA! THAT SHOULDER STRENGTHENING GAME IS ON POINT!"

That's the difference. I steadily began complimenting myself for the physical strength and flexibility exhibited by my body instead of denigrating it for not resembling pictures in magazines. When I started doling out high fives instead of going on "shade parades," I saw that I had a lot to be thankful for in my own body. My meaty thighs, once cast into shameful darkness because of their width and girth, proved to be secret weapons in my balance and standing posture practice. My chubby belly, once a constant source of embarrassment, began to give me a sense of pride because I was amazed by my ability to engage the surprisingly strong core muscles underneath. It seemed like a waste of time to hate these aspects of myself, when they were obviously key contributors to my overall strength and self-confidence.

In my opinion, the experience of practicing yoga at home and photographing the practice is a more genuine definition of the eight limbed path because it disregards the opinions of others that can become overbearing in a classroom environment. In a group class, the opinions of both teachers and fellow students have a tendency to distract even the most devoted yoga practitioners. Photographing a home practice is an opportunity to reclaim the strength that can be mutilated by the opinions of others.

For me, it doesn't matter if the superficial Western yoga world ever truly accepts and promotes the curvy, black female body. After all, it's not as though any other aspect of our whitewashed society has openly accepted fat, black women en masse. My only concern is making sure that my fat black sisters understand that yoga is for them, regardless of what society wants them to think. Prior to apps like Instagram and blogging platforms like Tumblr, Western marketing ploys were designed specifically to harvest body dissatisfaction in pursuit of monetary gain. However, with the advent of social media, we finally have a platform for exploring the actual body dissatisfaction imbedded in all humans. And, in response, "beauty centric" marketing ploys are under scrutiny. The progress toward change may be slow, but it is critical to note that it would be even slower coming without the influence of a robust and active online community.

Every day, whether it's via social media or real life interactions with my yoga students, I encounter brand-new diverse bodied yoga practitioners who cite the Instagram yoga community as the origin of their practice. People of all gender expressions, lifestyles, and bodily handicap are building yoga practices that reflect the unique edges of their everyday lives. Because social media offers both autonomy and community, there's a remarkable number of people who have chosen to document their physical practice for the same reasons that fueled my early Instagram presence. The proof of change is evident in a multitude of areas, including the rise of plus-size active wear options and the growing ubiquity of yoga classes specifically directed toward various marginalized communities. In many ways, the "body-positive" phrase has become a trendy and potentially misunderstood label. As one would expect, change has come about slowly and there are dissenting opinions within the body-positivity movement about how best to seek equality.

Ultimately, social media has redistributed a power dynamic once fully controlled by corporate media. Against the odds, the opportunity for an egalitarian yoga community is finally on the table. We now have a way to communicate with one another and form a utopian yoga community where all bodies are created equal—even fat, black ones. Maybe I'm too optimistic, but I think the online yoga world is the key to evolution within the "real" yoga world. By manually carving space for diverse bodied yoga practitioners online, we can usher in a new generation of yoga practitioners who see yoga's eight limbed path for what it truly is—the great equalizer and unifier of all humanity.

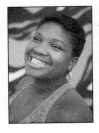

Jessamyn Stanley is a North Carolina–based yoga teacher and writer, and the creator of Cody App's EveryBody Yoga. Her blog and Instagram offer body positive advice for yoga practitioners and attract thousands of followers daily. Stanley has been featured by a wide range of international and national media outlets including *Good Morning America*, *Al Jazeera English*, *New York Magazine*, *The Huffington Post*, *The Daily Mail*, and *The Sunday Times*, among others.

Author photo by Zoe Litaker.

# WHOSE YOGA IS IT ANYWAY?: AN INDIAN AMERICAN'S ADVENTURES IN YOGALAND

## *Lakshmi Nair*

Yoga was exploding in Denver in 2005. I had just returned to the United States from a three-year sojourn in India, where I studied yoga at Vivekananda Yoga Kendra and Kaivalyadhama Ashram. I thought those conditions seemed ripe for me to start teaching yoga. Yet, for some reason, it just wasn't clicking for me. I wasn't attracting a following and at a pay rate of $3/student, I wasn't even making enough to cover gas. My mind slipped into a constant loop of negative self-talk.

"You are no good at this ... People just don't like you ... You aren't glamorous enough ... You don't have a yoga body ... You can't do advanced poses ... Face it, you stink ... Just give up and get a real job."

Just as I was about to throw in the yoga towel, I was given an opportunity to teach a yoga class for women of color. Being in that room with them for the first time, I exhaled. A softness spread through my center and then this truth bubbled to the surface: Of course! How could I teach yoga when I couldn't even breathe?

# My "Yoga Story"

Often in American yoga settings, we are asked to tell our "yoga story" —how we came to yoga. Invariably most of the stories start with asana...perhaps a humorous anecdote about trying to get a leg behind the head followed by a sense that there's "something deeper" which then ignites into a full-blown yoga passion. My yoga story doesn't begin with asana. Asana came much later. Being from a fairly religious South Indian Hindu family growing up in suburban Colorado, my introduction to yoga was through cassette tapes and comic books. Devotional songs (and film songs) were the soundtrack of my childhood. My introduction to the wisdom and philosophy of yoga came through my treasured collection of Amar Chitra Katha comic books gifted to me by my grandfather. These comics are beautifully illustrated stories from the *Puranas*, the epics, the *Upanishads*, Indian history, and folklore. As my first taste of representation in reading material, I devoured them hungrily. Until then, I didn't know how badly I was starving to see people who looked like me and reflected the culture of my family. I couldn't get enough. I would read and re-read the ones I had until their pages grew tattered. Every time I went to India (to this day), I would betray my American privilege by buying a stack of thirty or forty at once.

What I absorbed and assimilated from these stories is that my culture (at least our pre-colonial culture) prized spirituality over materialism. They told tale after tale of people rejecting the material world to seek God, demonstrating compassion by seeing God in all beings, and devoting the simplest acts of everyday life to the Divine. There was a heck of a lot of yoga in those stories, including asana (which is why I really bristle when I hear people claim that asana is actually European in origin). These stories instilled in me a tremendous love and pride in my cultural heritage.

During my teenage years, my father exposed me to meditation and asana. He decided I needed to learn traditional discipline and he would wake me up at 4:30 a.m. (yes, 4:30 a.m.!!) to do one hour of asana and half an hour of meditation. My teenage meditations were half hour snoozes.

Thus I looked forward to meditation and dreaded asana with every ounce of my being.

In college, believing I should be the "tolerant Hindu," I gave up my practice for the comfort of my Born Again Christian roommate. I only rediscovered yoga again in my late twenties when my life was in total shambles. And that time, it began with an asana class at Integral Yoga Ashram in San Francisco. It reconnected me to my roots and to my body, with which I had completely lost touch. I grew to love asana and to respect its power. Being in the (pre-gentrified) Mission district, the class was very diverse, and though I was often confused and amused by the teacher's pronunciation of Sanskrit names, I never felt awkward or out of place in the class. In fact, I felt really connected because this stuff was in my bones and my blood. Re-centered, I found the strength to leave the abusive marriage in which I found myself bound.

I decided to go to India to pursue formal study of yoga and to further connect to my roots and my spirituality. After three years, I came back to Colorado with a baby and an Indian husband in tow ... my *Eat, Pray, Love* story before *Eat, Pray, Love* was a thing!

Upon my return from India, I tried to jump into American private yoga studio culture and I found myself constantly in a state of existential crisis. It was odd and depressing to try to fit myself into this hole that was shaped so very differently from everything I thought was yoga. Attempting to stuff myself into clinging synthetic spandex that would take me a year of teaching yoga to pay for with my top heavy, post-natal midsection suffocating my face in *sarvangasana* as all those smiling skinny white women on the covers of yoga magazines ocked me from the grocery store checkout stands was a little bit of a self-esteem killer. I thought the point of yoga was to be conscious of the Self, not self-conscious!

What did it mean that I was teaching classes that I couldn't afford to take? The commercialism and high pricing, which in turn leads to an elitist and homogenous yoga culture disturbed me. In the precious stories of my childhood, yoga was a spiritual tradition and it wasn't free, but it was based on respectful exchange and faith in the spiritual principle of *karma*. I thought of my paternal grandfather, who was an Ayurvedic physician. He would accept payment in fish from fisherman even though he and his entire family were strict vegetarians. And yet he was one of the first in the town of Trivandrum to own a car. He was well off because those who could paid him with respect according to their means. Yoga is oft touted as a 6 billion dollar business in the West. Meanwhile, some studios were paying me $3/student to teach. How is it yogic if all this money is being made from yoga but teachers are being exploited rather than respected and cared for and expected to compete in a popularity contest for students?

And there was the surreal stuff: like when my Indian body entered a yoga space, I was either greeted with googly eyes as if I were the Goddess Lakshmi Herself descended from the heavens and any words I uttered were instantly magical and profound OR I was greeted with defensiveness as if my presence made people feel they had to prove their knowledge of Sanskrit, yoga, and all things Indian. Both of these attitudes made it very hard for me to just show up as a person. I felt like I was expected to be an enlightened yogini just because I'm Indian. I'm not enlightened. I'm not a yogi. To me, the word "yogi" refers to people who renounce material life to live in an ashram or a cave and devote their entire lives to the practice of yoga. I live in the world. I like donuts and Netflix and I have student loans. (And somehow I suspect that even if I changed my name to Satyanandamayi Ma and moved to a Himalayan mountaintop, Sallie Mae would still find me). I, like most everyone else I know, am just a *yogabhyasi*, "one who practices yoga," not a *yogi*, "one who has realized the state of yoga."

Everywhere I looked, I was nowhere to be found. All the South Asian flavor in yoga had been reduced to bindis and henna and Ganesha on spandex (on skinny white ladies). I hear people of color say they don't do yoga because yoga is a white lady thing. Heck, even I think it's a white lady thing, and, as an Indian, that is a real downer! Yoga is one of the most beautiful aspects of my heritage, yet we have been thrust into yoga's ancient past and totally left out of yoga's present. Yoga philosophy itself states that yoga is a universal truth that belongs to none and is accessible to all AND cultural appropriation is a thing. It exists much the same way that Disney can make a movie about the Little Mermaid, and it can be really, really popular, but it's still a bastardization of the beautiful, complex and deep Hans Christian Andersen fairy tale. That's not to say there aren't plenty of good folk out there who know and prefer the original. But that doesn't change the fact that most people you meet only know the Disney YogaLand version.

## The Last Straw: Yoga Racism

While romanticization of our culture might seem preferable to outright bigotry and ignorance, I feel a lump in my throat chakra when I hear white folks singing the praises of Rama, a Hindu God who is said to be an avatar of Vishnu, one of the trinity of Hindu patriarchal deities and is the hero of the epic *Ramayana*. Do I bring up that Desi (South Asian) feminists revile Rama for his treatment of his wife Sita (though She Herself is an avatar of the Goddess Lakshmi) and risk getting flooded with those pitying looks that I get when I wear a bindi (the mark worn traditionally by Hindu women on the third eye chakra point)... hip on white women, but a marker of patriarchal oppression on me? Do I bring up the Dravidian nationalist theory that the *Ramayana* is a narrative of Aryan colonization of the Dravidian South in which the Dravidians are rendered as monkeys and demons?

I can hear the whoosh of air going over people's heads. Do I mention that of all the millions of Hindu gods, Rama is the most beloved icon of Hindu nationalists, who are a dangerously Islamophobic, patriarchal, fascist group who wield considerable political power in India today. Rama is to today's India as Trump's/Pence's Jesus is to today's America, an unforgiving icon of intolerance and misogyny. When in modern India, Hindu fundamentalists are actively appropriating yoga, yoking it to the most oppressive and intolerant aspects of Indian culture, it does South Asians no favors when Western yogis unwittingly glorify their narrative. Do I mention that Bhakti yoga was actually a medieval spiritual rebellion against the oppressive hierarchies of casteism and patriarchal power and not a rave party? For me, as a South Asian feminist *yogabhyasi*, to be able to come to a place of true authenticity in my relationship to yoga, it's essential for me to examine all the historical complexities and to attempt to untangle the deeply interwoven threads of patriarchy and casteism. But when everything about yoga is mystified, potentially negative aspects are rendered invisible or, worse, made sacrosanct.

What finally made me want to give up on yoga teaching for good was when being the only person of color at a fund raiser ironically for yoga in "urban" schools, I became an "invisible" witness to culturally insensitive stereotyping of black people, couched in feel-good "yoga-speak." That was the last straw. I decided I just couldn't be a part of YogaLand anymore. I felt battered by this egoistic yoga that was like beauty standards … externally defined by a capitalist, patriarchal, racist framework that leaves everyone—even the skinny white women it puts up on a pedestal—out in the spiritual cold.

But as *dharma* would have it, that is when I was offered an opportunity to teach a yoga class for Women of Color.

## We Need a Safe Space

The Center for Trauma and Resilience (formerly Denver Center for Crime Victims), founded by a woman of color, offers a trauma sensitive yoga program to various affinity groups, including Women of Color. Their program recognized that just being a person of color in American society is traumatic! Cue ray of light streaming through cloud break and chorus of angels! I was the teacher, but I needed that safe space just as much as the participants in that room did. No wonder I had failed so miserably at connecting with people! I had never allowed myself to drop into a true place of authenticity. I was always worried about how my brown body was being perceived … as too unfit, too basic, too Indian, not Indian enough, etc. I could relate to the discomfiting space my students land in when they attempt to connect with their bodies in a homogenous yoga culture that renders their bodies invisible and yet hyper visible at the same time. I understood the futility of trying to unravel chronic embedded trauma in a space that is triggering. But here in this safe space, we could reclaim our bodies. We could let down our defenses and give the parasympathetic nervous system its turn to do the restorative and healing work that is so needed and too often eclipsed in a society in which our bodies and being aren't valued.

Isn't Yoga for People of Color segregation? Isn't it unyogic if we are supposed to be "all one" and beyond race and gender? Inclusivity and safe space are not at odds with each other. They are just two different fronts of the same struggle to make the world a better place. Alice Walker describes this concept best when she defines the term *Womanist* as one who is "committed to the survival and wholeness of the entire people, male and female. Not a separatist, except periodically, for health." Safe space allows us to acknowledge and heal the trauma of living in a racist society by arming us with effective, health-promoting tools to maneuver through a world that is stacked against us. But it doesn't mean we are any less committed to the wholeness and healing of the entire world. In fact, our lives, more than those with privilege, depend on it.

## Yoga Teacher Training for People of Color

I watched these women in my Women of Color class sink into deep *savasana* and I wanted to cry. The participants were so warm and appreciative and they restored my faith in yoga and in myself. I realized that the demand for POC yoga was so much greater than the supply of teachers. I took a leap and decided to start my own yoga immersion/teacher training for people of color, with the intention of increasing the diversity of the yoga teacher pool in Denver, but equally importantly to give people of color a safe space to really dive in deep … to explore and heal the physical, mental, emotional, and spiritual wounds of oppression using the powerful tools of yoga. It also allows me to reclaim yoga as an indigenous healing wisdom tradition with authenticity, where I can feel free to be real about the good, the bad, and the ugly of yoga … where I can bring my whole self and my students can bring their whole selves too.

## "Talking About the Negative Is What Has Been Positive"

In my teacher training, when we talk about the root chakra, we dig deep into the historical traumas of slavery, genocide, colonization, war, and the impacts those things have on our bodies and our being. We talk about daily assaults and threats to our physical safety and security due to police brutality, economic structural racism, hate crimes, and war. When we speak about the solar plexus chakra and body issues and self-esteem, we speak about the lack of representation of our bodies in the media and all the macro- and microaggressions that assault every aspect of our bodies and self-esteem—our skin, our hair, our noses. How even our names and the markers of our identities (clothing, hair, language, etc.) are often violently or subtly stripped from us. When we talk about the heart chakra, we are allowed to express our profound grief for Sandra Bland, Tamir Rice, the children of Flint, the thousands of unaccompanied minors crossing the border, Syrian refugees, and the ever increasing tally of lives that don't matter in our current system. We explore what forgiveness looks like when it isn't thrust upon us or expected from us.

In homogenous yoga settings, these kind of conversations are often seen as political (hence, not spiritual) or negative. But people of color simply don't have the luxury of viewing the world through rose-colored YogaLand glasses. For us, enlightenment means seeing what is, even if it isn't pretty. As one of my students said, "The discussion on darkness as a place of beauty and healing, I think, is core to why our group works. Talking about the negative is what has been positive."

## Backlash

This movement to create safe, healing space comes at a perfect time too, given our current political climate. The tide of the Civil Rights movement is again rising with *#BlackLivesMatter*. And along with that, the backlash against all people of color is growing stronger too, sadly even in spaces where we naively presumed we would be met with compassion, as we saw this year with people of color yoga in Seattle and elsewhere. Hate and yoga should be like oil and water, but somewhere, to make it more marketable, we have thrown in an emulsifier. It is curious to me that no other affinity group raises as much ire and violent opposition as people of color. Instead of asking us why we need separate space, perhaps the questions should be more introspective. *Svadhyaya* (self-study) is, after all, one of the essential eight limbs of yoga. Like the parable of the blind friends and the elephant, how much depth and richness of understanding is an insular and homogenous yoga community missing out on? How can this be shifted toward genuine inclusivity that feels safe for all? How can the larger yoga community extend its tremendous resources to support and protect yoga for people of color in this heated climate?

## Human Beings Must Create Peace

As the Dalai Lama famously said,[1] "Peace does not come through prayer, we human beings must create peace." When people of color take the lead in our own healing, we dig deep into the heart of the problems of our world. The Ego's separation from Self, which causes all of our individual suffering, is the very same separation mentality that creates all the suffering in the world and POC bodies are a *kshetra* (field) upon which this mentality is enacted. This is why the first Indian gurus to come West like Swami Vivekananda and Paramahamsa Yogananda were spiritually called here to share yoga. By no coincidence, they came at the height of the Indian anti-colonial movement. Yoga was meant to be an antidote to the mentality that created colonialism. POC, or any other kinds of affinity group yoga, should not be seen as an affront to yogic values. We cannot strive to liberate ourselves alone. To truly free ourselves from suffering, we must work tirelessly to end the suffering of every being on the planet, because we are all One. That is our *dharma*. Yoga IS social justice.

---

1. "Quotes from HH The Dalai Lama," Zen Moments. February 20, 2017. Accessed June 11, 2017. https://zenmoments.org/dalai-lama-quotes/.

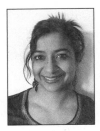

Lakshmi Nair is a yoga teacher based in Denver, Colorado. She teaches trauma sensitive yoga for the Center for Trauma and Resilience and is the founder of Satya Yoga Immersion and Yoga Teacher Training for People of Color. The three sacred intentions of her work are to make the teachings of yoga truly universal and accessible to all peoples, to offer a safe space for people of color to address the effects of racism and oppression on our bodies, minds, and spirits using the healing tools provided by yoga, and to put a little bit of India back into yoga.

Author photo by Arun Lakshman.

# THE RAPUNZEL GAME

## *Dr. Sabrina Strings*

There's a cute new form of segregation taking the yoga world by storm. Here's how I found out about it: I was attending a yoga teacher training during the fall of 2013 and one of our teachers was an affable hippie named Mimi. Mimi had spent several decades training with, and subsequently teaching, yoga practitioners in the San Francisco Bay Area. She was leading a meditation workshop as one of our monthly day-long intensives. About midway through our seven-hour slog, she sensed our restlessness and exhaustion. She was encouraged to switch things up a bit.

"Get into groups of two," she advised.

I turned to see that the woman sitting next to me was Amy. Amy was an African-American woman with a perm and a bourgeois manner. I had diagnosed Amy with people of color blindness.[1] This is a condition in which people of color—often black—embrace the America-is-colorblind discourse. They subsequently refuse to *see* other people of color—often black—and avoid interactions with them in an ironic and

---

1. This term is an homage to Jared Sexton's "people-of-color-blindness." However, while I am using the term to describe the phenomenon in which black people literally do not want to see other black people, Sexton uses the term to articulate a racial politics in which liberals purport that all persons of color have similar experiences of oppression under white supremacy, ignoring the "specificity of anti-blackness" in the United States (2010: 48).

assimilationist attempt to pretend as if there is, indeed, nothing to be seen. Of course underlying this behavior is the fear that someone will see them and recognize that they are, in fact, *black.*

Amy and I had never been in a group together. In reality, Amy rarely made eye contact with me. She usually gave my mat a wide berth when she was deciding where to place hers. On the day in question, she placed her mat next to mine while I was in the bathroom, thus wholly unaware that someone would see the two black women sitting together in the training, and put two and two together.

When Mimi announced that we needed to find partners, I immediately went on the offensive. Sharon, the quirky but inscrutable white lady in front of me would make a good partner, so I lunged forward to tap her shoulder. Too late—someone else had already snapped Sharon up.

"Do you want to be partners?" Amy asked. I froze mid-lunge, slowly bringing my hips back to my heels. I looked over to confirm that she did, in fact, mean me. She did.

"Uhhhhhh, sure."

Mimi continued her with instructions.

"After you have chosen your partner, just sit in silence for a moment." She took a beat, giving the yogis a chance to settle in to their dyads.

"Okay, when you open your eyes, I'd like you to tell your partner about your experience with meditation since you started the training. How often are you practicing? What has been your experience sitting? Have you incorporated meditation into your regular yoga routine? If not, what barriers do you have to making it a regular part of your practice." She paused, allowing us to digest this information. Then she added,

"And I'd like the woman with the shortest hair to go first."

My head shot up, mouth agape. I looked from Mimi to Amy. Mimi was oblivious, concerning herself with preparations for the next assignment. Amy had a half-smile playing around the corners of her mouth. She raised her eyebrows and parted her lips expectantly, a mute expression of superiority that said, *that means you.*

It was amazing nobody got shanked.

I wasn't about to argue the point with Amy. Instead, while she sat with one eyebrow cocked, I settled back in to my meditation. Occasionally, I'd open my mouth to respond to one of the questions Mimi had posed and then return to silence. When it was Amy's turn to go, I maintained my meditative posture, completely tuning her out. The exercise, and whatever it was supposed to help us learn from one another, was a wash.

I was at a loss. This type of comparison seemed curiously out of place, given my yoga experience up to that point. I'd found yoga four years prior. I took my first class on a lark, tapering as I was from a serious running habit. But, over the course of those four years, I kept coming back because it gave me the tools to feel comfortable in my own skin. Being a black woman in America, there were many times in which I felt reviled, unwanted, because I was seen as physically different from the white "norm." Yoga helped me discover my internal power and beauty. It was a form of liberation.

I'd listened attentively as teachers preached about self-love, tolerance, and the unity of all beings. Of course, the yoga community wasn't perfect. There were many times when my racial difference was marked, when people would move their mat from mine, trying to articulate some false colorblind explanation ("Oh, there's more space over there…"). But before Mimi made us play this hair game, I could not remember a time when difference was purposefully called out, brought to the fore, used to divide. I could not think of another time in which we were called to order ourselves based on physical appearance.

There were a couple of reasons I was disappointed that Mimi made us mark the difference, made us play what I'm calling "the Rapunzel Game." For one, this game invited "comparing mind." Comparing mind is the innate tendency for all humans to compare themselves to others. These comparisons can be based on anything. But they are often based on things that have a social or economic value (e.g., how much money you earn, how you look, the area where you live), and can engender hierarchies between persons or groups. In contemplative practice communities, we are encouraged to let these types of comparisons go.

Second, and relatedly, the Rapunzel Game invites an invidious *racialized* and gendered form of comparing mind. Long straight hair, and short curly hair, have had clear social values attached to them in Western culture due to their respective associations with whiteness and blackness.

Indeed, the sorting of people based on the length—and relatedly the texture—of their hair dates back to slavery.[2] With the onset of the slave trade during the fifteenth century, artists and philosophers routinely compared the newly encountered African women to European women. By the sixteenth century, as the judgments of black women became more derisive, these comparisons were used to reify European superiority. Black women's hair was often at the center of these assessments. The long, straight, blond hair of deified Roman goddess Venus was the gold standard; black women's curly locks were deemed inferior.

By the seventeenth century, comparisons of black and white hair would become a lynchpin of scientific racism. The first man to ever draft a racial hierarchy made the appearance of African hair integral to his classification schema, writing, "... their hair is not truly hair but instead a sort of wool"(Bernier 2001: 248). Indeed, by this era, the stereotype that Africans had short hair—which, because it was unlike Europeans', wasn't truly hair at all—was a well-worn invective (Kolfin 2010).

As African slaves made their way to the United States, hair was a pivotal marker of race and status (Tharps 2009). Along with lighter skin, straighter, longer hair could give slaves access to "better food, living conditions and a chance at an otherwise illegal education" (Tharps 2009). It was within this cultural milieu that the term "good hair," meaning hair that is straight or with looser curl pattern, was born and circulated among African Americans (Tharps 2009).

It wasn't until the 1960s that black people mounted a significant challenge to this hegemonic aesthetic. The Black Power movement in particular rejected the reliance on white (long and straight) hair and

---

2. With the revival of classical ideals during the Renaissance, Venus, the Roman goddess of love, came to represent the epitome of beauty. She was praised, amongst other things, for her long flaxen hair (Schreuder and Kolfin 2008).

beauty ideals, urging people to get rid of straighteners and wear their hair in its natural state. (Angela Davis and her massive natural became formidable and iconic symbols of black resistance.) Many black people, impacted by the critical social movements of the era, wore their hair in Afros, reclaiming a sense of pride in their coils.

But, the pride and protest of the social movements of the previous generation did not overturn long-standing hegemonic ideals by which women in the West (regardless of race) are still being judged. There remains a hierarchy of beauty in these United States. The women sitting at the top have these qualities: White or light skin with long, straight blond hair.[3]

A simple perusal of the fashion and beauty magazines at your local drug store will reveal the obviousness of the truth. Whether it's Blake Lively or Jennifer Lawrence or Jennifer Aniston or any number of the celebrities perched atop the mountain of mainstream ideals, many, many will fit the mold. Most may have died their hair, straightened it, grown it out, or bought extensions because they know that straight, long blond hair can be a tremendous asset. However they arrive, as if inspired by Rapunzel, they cultivate this style because of the seeming opportunities for social and economic prosperity this hair affords them.

I didn't say any of this to Mimi, and I did my best to meet Amy where she was. As a yoga and meditation practitioner living in the Bay Area, Mimi would undoubtedly have claimed to be concerned about social justice. All the while, she was blissfully unaware of how her actions in the studio participated in a system of sorting rooted in slavery.

At the time, I dismissed the "game" as a one-off. I thought it was a peculiar if annoying sorting tool she thought fit to deploy. I was wrong.

The following year, I enrolled in another yoga and meditation training. On the first day of this training, the Rapunzel Game resurfaced. This time it was "And let the person with the *longest* hair go first!" Later that same day, this game was played again, "And the person with the *shortest* hair should go first!" That last time, my partner in the game,

---

3. I would also add that these women are usually thin and blue-eyed, qua the Nordic/Aryan ideal rigorously promoted in this country between the 1890s–1930s (Strings 2012).

who had straight hair, asked why don't we unwrap our buns (and I would also have to unravel my twists) to compare lengths?

I noticed there was a titillated sense of glee in playing this game, specifically among women with straight, long hair. In fact, in the many times I was forced to play this game, *every single time* it was proposed by a woman with straight or wavy, long hair.

At this training, I decided to take it up with the staff. I sent a note to the one black person on the team, Jesse. She was not a regular faculty member—all of the faculty were white—but an assistant. I explained to her that I was offended by the Rapunzel Game. I had noticed that some of the older women with short hair were visibly irritated, and I imagined the game was less than fun for balding men.

"Unless being in a yoga training now requires black women to get perms," I said, "I'm not sure how I'm supposed to measure the length of my hair." It was, moreover, unclear how that was supposed to add to my spiritual advancement. I asked her if I was imagining that this game was offensive and racially biased. She replied, "No, I felt that too."

Jesse relayed our grievance to the faculty. They expressed heartfelt concern. Issued an apology to the entire training, claiming that the game exposed an unconscious form of white privilege. This was close, but no cigar. Having straight, long hair is not inherently a "privilege." Its value has had a good deal to do with its historical link to whiteness in a society that has made comparisons based on hair and deemed this type superior. In this way, it reveals itself not as an example of white privilege but an example of white supremacy.

I had hoped that was the end of it. It wasn't. One year later, same training, new faculty, the Rapunzel Game made a comeback. This time it was started by Carter, a multiracial woman, with long, wavy hair. When I confronted her about it, she became defensive. Said there was nothing wrong with short hair. Many people are proud to have short hair. This was of course, beside the point. I, like many black naturals, love my hair. I love it long, I love it short. Its kink and swirl makes me feel like an original. It's full of body and life. This, however, doesn't mean I had escaped being measured against white ideals of beauty, telling me how my hair should look (hint: long and straight). I'd had to re-sist dominant hair narratives to find what was best for me.

Though she was herself part black, and looked to be in her forties, Carter had apparently missed the social movements asserting pride in various African hair textures and lengths, and had never heard any de-risive statements being made about black women's hair (not even those by Don Imus.) She reminded me of dear, POC-blind Amy. She told me, in no uncertain terms, "I think hair *is* race and gender neutral."

Whether or not something is racially biased is not based on a straw poll of the available people of color. It is rooted in the historical and ongoing fact of domination. Short or long hair may have different meanings in different contexts, in other cultures. But in this country, we cannot conveniently sidestep the historical *and current* meaning attached to straight, long (and often blond) hair.

The Rapunzel Game is more than a racially biased pastime that sev-eral people I have encountered find strange and offensive. It serves as an important reminder of the fact that despite many yoga studios' best ef-forts, the space they are holding may feel neither safe nor welcoming for those persons who are not in (or unlike Amy and Carter, do not aspire to resemble) the majority. In yoga, the majority are white and female. Several news articles have pointed to the overwhelming whiteness and femininity of modern yoga. For most, the question is about the cause (i.e., "how did we get here?"). Questions about the consequences of yoga being largely white and female are rarely considered. And yet the consequences are significant. One consequence is that women of color, men of all backgrounds, and queer or trans persons may enter a space that claims to be inclusive but feels hostile.

If yoga studios truly are invested in creating safe and inclusive spaces for the motley crew of potential practitioners, it would behoove them to end games that require people to sort themselves based on physical difference. Should we organize people by weight next time? Thinnest people go first? Or how about height? Shortest people go first? Or eye color, blue eyes go first?

Games that require practitioners to point out differences, measure them, discuss them, then *order* themselves based on these differences are not only slow and inefficient sorting mechanisms. They also invite the comparing mind that we are supposed to be checking at the door. And—even if unintentionally—they pick up on the necessarily racialized and sexualized legacy-creating hierarchies based on physical appearance. A tip for teachers: just let the group members decide who goes first.

I took these trainings hoping to be able to extend the yoga wisdom, to adapt the skills I learn, and to deliver them to underserved communities. I've learned a lot about what goes on in yoga, not all of it for the best. The Rapunzel Game and countless other instances of oppressive and exclusionary practices in yoga are what motivate me to continue to examine and critique current practices and to cultivate an awareness that can make our practice feel more like it belongs to all of us.

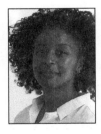

Sabrina Strings, PhD, is an assistant professor of Sociology at UC Irvine and a 200-hour CYT. Her work is featured in *Yoga International*, *The Feminist Wire*, *Feminist Media Studies*, and *Signs: Journal of Women in Culture and Society*. She is also the cofacillitator of the Race and Yoga Working Group at UC Berkeley.

Author photo by Heather Ashbach, UCI.

# SO WE CAN BREATHE

## *Chanelle John*

Learning to love my body has been one of the most significant things I've accomplished. Growing up as a black girl in America, I knew self-love was never a given. Black was beautiful in my house, with portraits of black dancers and jazz musicians hung on the walls. Messages that conflicted with joy and affirmation I felt at home were everywhere. There weren't many black families in my childhood town, leaving me feeling conspicuous and isolated. When I turned on the TV or opened a magazine, I rarely saw girls like me or women who looked who I'd become.

The media I consumed as a child conveyed Eurocentric beauty standards in no uncertain terms: thin and white, preferably with flowing hair. I was black, and my hair was usually defying combs and gravity, plaited with braids and beads. The lack of representation for women of color left me feeling alienated. The media messages taught me, and millions of other girls, that the pinnacle of beauty was being white and slim, and the goal of womanhood was to be beautiful. This sexist, white supremacist beauty ideal poisoned my self-image.

Magazines and movies insist that if we buy certain products, eat certain foods, and act a certain way, we too can conform to beauty norms and be successful. But this beauty standard is intentionally nearly impossible to achieve, leaving girls feeling inferior in its shadow. This can engender a sense of shame, hopelessness, and worthlessness. When girls and women internalize the beauty norms, it can mean being at war with our body image—especially for girls of color.

I internalized this dissonance until it morphed my view of myself. I slowly became more and more preoccupied with my weight, evolving into what I would later learn was body dysmorphia. It grew worse as I got older, quickly developing hips and thighs that belied my age. I resented my body and treated it like a problem to correct, an obstacle that I needed to overcome. Eventually this resentment and body dysmorphia led to cycles of disordered eating. I was either restricting my food and overexercising or binging and purging. Middle school, high school, and college found me vacillating between those two extremes.

In 2011, after years of body dysmorphia and disorder eating, I started therapy and realized that it was possible to break free from my struggles with body image. Therapy helped me change my habits, but therapy alone couldn't heal the chasm between my body and mind. I knew that there was work I had to do on myself, that no therapist or counselor could do for me. I had to get in touch with my body's needs and redefine health for myself.

## Rediscovering Intuition

I deeply wanted to be healthy but I didn't understand what life-long health entailed. The images I saw in media and magazines taught me that health was fad diets, fat phobia, and relentless exercise. I decided to limit my exposure to that toxic "health" paradigm, and the beauty standard it promotes. I cancelled my subscriptions to exercise magazines and became much more discerning about the media I consumed. Instead of following generalized dieting and exercise advice, I committed to using my intuition when it came to my health. Meditation helped me cultivate the self-awareness I needed to understand and respond to my body's needs. Radical self-acceptance and compassion became the tools that helped me heal my relationship to my body. Only then did I see that food was fuel for my body and not just a tool for weight control. I created a body-positive, shame free relationship to fitness and transformed my yoga practice in the process.

When I first discovered yoga in my early teens, I wrangled the expansive beautiful tradition into my flawed fitness framework. My practice was a place of destruction instead of healing, constantly criticizing my body and trying to push myself further. While in therapy, my new yoga practice reemerged from my interest in meditation and mindfulness. As I read about the other limbs of yoga and it's spiritual principles, I realized I needed to start my practice from a place of non-harming, contentment, and surrender. Instead of setting lofty goals for extensive daily practices, I started small—one sun salutation a morning before I sat to meditate. Slowly, one day at a time, a new practice grew intuitively from a base of self-compassion. As I found yoga videos with incredible instructors like Seane Corn, my home practice became my haven. I learned to love my body and myself as it was instead of constantly comparing it to unrealistic beauty norms. I felt myself get stronger and my meditation practice persisted. Eventually, I got up the courage to practice at a yoga studio.

## Studio Struggles

It was difficult to find a yoga studio that fit. Getting up the nerve to walk through the door to one sometimes felt like an achievement unto itself. My initial experiences in yoga studios prodded the body image issues that I had been working through. By the time I entered my first studio class, I'd begun to heal my relationship to my body, but it was difficult. Every studio visit felt like a test of my progress.

I tried to make my curvy brown body invisible by wearing all black clothes and placing my mat near the back of the class. The media would have you believe that yoga is the sole province of lithe white women, and my studio experience mirrored that portrayal. I was regularly the only person of color in my classes. Sometimes I left the studio on a yoga cloud from my practice. Other times I felt defeated after being beside all the other yogis who were bold enough to practice in their sports bras. I wondered, *Can I really practice with all of these women who look like yoga models? Do I belong here?*

I also wrestled with another question: Can I even afford to be here? Yoga's commodification in the West has made it an exclusive pastime. The price of a class or even introductory offer is out of reach for so many people. Often I was one of them. When I first entered a yoga studio I had two jobs, but the majority of my money was dedicated to keeping my rent paid. Discretionary funds weren't easy to come by. Still, I diligently searched for deals and community classes to ensure I could practice in a studio. I persevered in my studio practice, but it wasn't easy. I let myself take child's pose whenever I needed without judgment and listened to my body as much as I did the instructor. I went to smaller classes with noncompetitive atmospheres, where I eventually felt comfortable moving my mat toward the front of the room. The confidence I gained from my inner work was palpable. I was reaping the benefits of a compassionate, intuitive, shame-free yoga practice.

I wanted to bring my friends and for them to experience the healing potential of yoga. But I knew that, for all of my challenges showing up in a brown body at a yoga studio, other marginalized groups were absent as well. As I looked around my studio classes and talked to my friends I wondered, *Where are the LGBTQ folks?* Where were the differently abled and the fat positive yogis? Western yoga culture and community's inability to address the racism, classism, ageism, and ableism kept yoga homogenous. It also made yoga inaccessible to populations that needed it most. It became clear to me then that I had a yoga practice and a community but not a yoga community. I wanted to see a yoga class with yogis from across the spectrum of human diversity. If I couldn't bring my community to yoga, I was determined to bring yoga to them. Five years after my first studio class, my commitment to bringing yoga to communities of color collided with the inception of the Black Lives Matter Movement.

## We Can't Breathe

On August 9, 2014, as my yoga teacher training was drawing to a close, an unarmed Missouri teen named Michael Brown was shot and killed by a police officer. I remember coming home after yoga practice and dropping my mat bag on the floor only to open Facebook and find my timeline buzzing with the news. I fell to my knees as I read the details. Recent high school grad. Twelve shots fired. Body left for four hours in the street. I was devastated and shaken. I remember wondering, *Who will be next?*

The previous month was tumultuous, as the video of Eric Garner dying in an officer's choke hold entered the news cycle. Witnessing a father and husband gasping, "I can't breathe" was traumatic, as was the lack of accountability for his death. For many, Michael Brown's death widened the wound from the loss of Eric Garner. The trauma felt relentless as more cases of police brutality flooded the news and the list of victims grew.

I walked through the motions of my life, going to work and yoga each day. But I couldn't shake the anger and sadness. In my mind, I was thinking of Michael Brown, Eric Garner, and Tamir Rice. Tamir, a twelve-year-old killed by police in Cleveland, reminded me of the kids I taught in my community yoga classes.

At the time, I was teaching the class at a library in one of Boston's black neighborhoods. Every Saturday morning, I would lead kids and their families through simple yoga sequences. I loved seeing the kids every week, their hair braided or barber shop pristine, dimples punctuating their grins, child-sized high tops beside their yoga mats. But sometimes when I looked into their faces, I saw our collective vulnerability. My yoga students, like Tamir, were young, black, and living in underserved neighborhoods. I worried for the ones whose height would soon belie their age, turning their bodies into targets of suspicion and fear. Their faces were in my mind while we protested that fall.

We marched through the streets, chanting the names of boys who would never grow to adulthood and demanding justice. When I was feeling enraged, I would use my vinyasa practice to sweat it out on the mat. When tears gathered in my eyes, my practice was like a prayer, sending whatever grace I could to the victims' families and the protesters. I mourned for the female victims of police violence whose names were much more likely to be in my timeline than a headline. When I was overwhelmed by endless stories of black women's lives lost, I would close my computer and my eyes, place my hands on my heart and breathe. Focusing on the rise and fall of my chest, I breathed for Eric Garner, Michael Brown, Tamir Rice, Aiyana Stanley-Jones, and all the others who would never breathe again.

That fall, a vision for my future coalesced. I wanted to be of service, to bring yoga to all corners of the hood, and affirm black life in my work. I was painfully aware of the reasons black and low-income communities could benefit from yoga. The ramifications of absorbing beauty norms, the burden of defying racist tropes, and the struggle of surviving in a society based on capitalism and white supremacy burdens the mental and physical health of the black community. I became more committed than ever to take my yoga teaching beyond the studio.

## Yoga and Diversity in Practice

In the months following Black Lives Matter's inception, I created POC Practice, a yoga class for people of color. It was important to me that I hold a space for people to come together and heal in light of the collective violence we face. I envisioned POC Practice years earlier while attending hip-hop yoga classes at local studios. Practicing sweaty vinyasa sequences with hip-hop music was incredible. Hip-hop is home to me, like a native tongue. But being the only person of color in those classes was no homecoming. The classes, mostly attended by white people, were in close proximity to elite and expensive universities in a segregated city. I wanted to create a hip-hop yoga experience that felt uplifting and could be enjoyed without reservation.

I began teaching POC Practice at an accessible community space in Boston's South End. The South End held a special significance for me. Formally a vibrant part of Black Boston, it had undergone waves of gentrification that forced black families, mine included, to far corners of the city. The all-levels, donation-based community class brought people of color from across the racial and ethnic spectrum, and of all sizes and shades, back to the South End.

That winter a white ally and I cofounded the Yoga Diversity Initiative (YDI). At YDI, we provide scholarships for yogis of color to attend yoga teacher trainings. Having more visible teachers of color is an important step in rectifying yoga's racial divide. As I stated in an article for

Decolonizing Yoga, "Despite the stunning array of options one has for a yoga teacher training, these programs are still certifying teachers that promote yoga's status quo. To effectively combat this image issue, and to teach to diverse communities in a culturally sensitive way, there will need to be more yoga instructors of color."[1]

While in their yoga teacher training, the yogis are paired with a mentor who is a yoga teacher of color. The scholarship recipients have built-in support for any racial, class, or other issues that may come up in their training. After the training, our awardees each teach a number of free classes in neighborhoods of color as *seva*, or selfless service. When we train and support yoga teachers of color and send them back out into their communities, we expand the idea of what a "yoga body" is. We affirm to them that they too can take part in this beautiful tradition. I hope that, by doing this work, people of color can experience the type of grounding and resilience that yoga has given me.

## *Yamas* and *Niyamas*: Keys to Transformation

There are many challenges to self-acceptance, body-positivity, and life-long health. I've seen firsthand the damage oppression does to our sense of self. I've spent years trying to unlearn sexist, unrealistic beauty standards I internalized. Deepening my understanding of yoga's non-physical aspects has become an invaluable part of my journey.

Yogic philosophy includes an ethical code, called the *yamas* and *niyamas*, that can help us transform our relationship to our yoga practice and ourselves. The yama *ahimsa* asks us to practice non-harming. Extending the gift of non-harming to ourselves can liberate us from constant self-criticism and judgment. *Satya*, or truthfulness, can help us interrogate the validity of the oppressive ideas we've internalized. The niyama *svadhyaya*, asks us to study and observe ourselves. Through compassionate and dedicated self-study, we can see the nuanced ways oppressive ideas hinder our relationships with ourselves and one another.

1. Chanelle John, "(More) Reasons Why Your Yoga Class Is So White," Decolonizing Yoga, August 28, 2014. Accessed August 15, 2017. http://www.decolonizingyoga.com/reasons-yoga-class-white/.

Through practicing the yamas and niyamas, we can reconnect with our intuition and separate who we are from what society tells us to be. It's rewarding to liberate ourselves from these limited notions of self, but it's a difficult process. Your intention to cultivate self-acceptance and self-love may run counter to years of conditioning and negative thought patterns. We must remember that we are worthy and that change is possible.

Though our bodies may appear different, we are all negatively impacted by oppressive ideologies. Sexism, racism, and sizeism impact the quality of all of our lives. They keep us from accepting our selves and divide us from one another. No matter what we look like, we all have something to gain from naming and dismantling these oppressive ideas and the systems they represent. With commitment, compassion, and bravery we can lift the burden of oppression so we, collectively, can breathe.

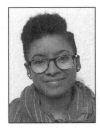

Chanelle John is a race scholar, yoga instructor, and business owner based in Boston, MA. Prior to completing her yoga teacher training, she received her BA from Goddard College, studying the intersections of racial identity, culture, and art. She can be found teaching at libraries and community groups in Boston, as well as online at www.wholesoulhealthco.com.

Author photo by Tatiana M. R. Johnson.

# PART 3 MOVING INWARD & UPWARD

- Why is accessibility in yoga important to you?
- Think of one way you've helped to shift the tide toward making yoga more inclusive.
- What are two ways you can support and participate in the movement to make yoga more body-positive and less exclusive?
- How do others benefit from your healing and how do you, in turn, benefit from the liberation of others?

# PART FOUR

## *Challenging Exclusivity and Creating Space*

Just as there isn't one style, form, or way to practice yoga, bodies that practice yoga are diverse and varied. On the surface, though, it may seem that yoga practice consists merely of asana, or physical postures (often, ones that seem to be available only to those with a genetic propensity to contortionism and/or serious upper body strength). To boot, the often but not always, lithe and bendy bodies practicing those postures have been dubbed "yoga bodies," to the exclusion of most.

Fortunately, thanks to the committed and passionate bands of advocates on the ground and on social media, shifts have been occurring. The stories in this section challenge existing norms and offer alternative perspectives. They also remind us why it is our duty to make yoga more accessible in whatever way we can, emphasizing the importance of pushing back against the larger culture that has created, and continues to re-create, unrealistic expectations in which only the few are represented to the exclusion of the masses.

Suzannah Neufeld not only rejects the "yoga body" but also the pressure many women feel to return to their "pre-baby body." She offers a call to action, one that encourages us to learn how to listen and learn to trust our bodies. Most importantly, though, she provides a renewed definition of the "love your body" mantra with the hope that yoga moves us into service.

Dana Smith reveals the damage that may be unintentionally caused when we are viewed as our body alone and learn our worth is measured by how well this body fits the given cultural ideal. Yoga not only offered Smith a new way to relate to and inhabit her body but also inspired her mission to share the nondiscriminatory practice of yoga and provide a platform for the various bodies that breathe and move on the mat.

To explore the concept of "the yoga body," well-known yoga blogger, Roseanne Harvey, accepted Sadie Nardini's challenge to get the much coveted and desired "yoga body" in twenty-one days. A social experiment of sorts, Harvey shares some of the surprising and thought-provoking insights gained along the way.

Lauren Eckstrom not only describes the powerful transformation yoga forged in her life and in relationship to her body but also the perilous ground one often treads as a public figure, even in "conscious" spaces such as the yoga community. Eckstrom encourages us to expose the ways in which privilege operates as the impetus to increase solidarity and create meaningful cultural change in which we are all seen and heard.

Solidarity and connection in community is exactly what Elizabeth Wojtowicz craved most. Attributing her lack of self-confidence and extreme shyness to her disability, Wojtowicz desired a place outside of her family in which to feel accepted and whole. Yoga not only offered a newfound relationship with her whole self but a mindful community of activists.

# YOGA AND THE PRE-BABY BODY

## Suzannah Neufeld

Ali MacGraw was my first yoga teacher.

In 1996, when I was seventeen and hospitalized for an eating disorder, Ali's yoga VHS tape was the only movement I was allowed, and I loved her with a religious devotion, waiting all day for our special half hour together. You may think of her as an actress, but I think of her as a glorious yogini, stretching and breathing on silky white sandy dunes. I thought I was just pulling one over on my doctors, getting in some extra calorie burning at the end of the day. What I actually got was a practice that would nourish me for the rest of my life.

When I left the hospital, the doctor wrote a list of things she thought might help me on the road to recovery—YOGA was first on the list, in all caps. Though I didn't recover for five more years, she was right. Yoga was the rope that I used to pull myself out of the abyss of self-hatred, confusion, and alienation from my body and humanity.

I'm skipping the details of how yoga helped my body image then because that story has been beautifully told by so many others. I remember being a teen with an eating disorder in the days before the Internet, and I had never heard anyone else's story. At my local bookstore, I would scan the shelves for the one eating disorder memoir, open it within another book so no one could see the cover, and connect furtively and passionately to the words within, to know I wasn't alone. Today, eating disorder stories and memoirs are everywhere. There are even subgenres of recovery stories—and the story of the young white woman using yoga as a path to healing is a standard in the canon.

I'm picking up my story much later, after a long, steadfast recovery, with what fascinates me now—how yoga keeps revealing new gifts with each passing year of practice. Yoga, once my tool for healing my eating disorder, is now facilitating healing in how I relate to my body in a whole new era of my life, one that feels lifetimes away from my diet-obsessed teenage years: becoming a mother.

## Becoming a Mother

After recovering from my eating disorder in my early twenties, I went on to become a psychotherapist and yoga teacher with a mission to share the healing path of recovery and yoga with others. I felt grateful that I had learned to "love my body" and "trust my body" and wanted to share that opportunity. I recognize now that a big privilege I had in learning to "love" and "trust" my body was that even after gaining weight in my recovery, I was still relatively thin and visibly fit.

At age thirty-one, I became pregnant for the first time and gained a considerable amount of weight—mostly because I was so nauseated that the only way to keep from throwing up was to have food in my mouth. I also felt too sick to move much, and my yoga practice changed wildly. No more vinyasas, bandhas, and binds—I had to slow down and focus more on breath and mindful presence, which were (and always are) a blessing to help calm my brain's chatter and connect me to my baby.

After my daughter was born, I trusted my body to find its set point at its own pace. I was so sleep-deprived and focused on creating my new family and figuring out how to balance time with baby, work, partner, and self that I didn't really think about my body shape. A few months later, I realized that I had lost none of the weight I had gained in pregnancy—in fact, I'd actually gained more. I felt deeply ashamed and confused, unsure if I really could trust my body or love it anymore. This was compounded by "concerned" messages from my health provider about me being "overweight." As a person who had been walking around with thin privilege my whole life, I got my first taste of what many face every day—how a visit to the doctor's office becomes an opportunity to be shamed. Worse, I felt ashamed of being ashamed—as a body image activist and feminist, what does it mean when you suddenly feel bad about your body?

Articles like "10 Reasons Breastfeeding Is Best" tell you that nursing makes you lose weight. Not always! Nursing is an appetite stimulant for me—never have I been so constantly hungry as I was during the first year of my kids' lives. I take very good care of my health with food and exercise—and I've learned that a nontrivial amount of extra weight is just what my body likes while, you know, growing humans. As I write this, I have been either pregnant or nursing for six years straight (and counting), and my body has never been the same weight and shape for more than a few months at a time.

## Yoga in My "New" Body

One wonderful side effect of the "baby weight" changes in my body is that I was forced to become a beginner again at yoga asana. After years of being able to do contortionist poses a la magazine covers (and, by the way, suffering in my low back for it), I now could barely touch my toes. I had to let go of fourteen years of practice and humbly begin building strength and flexibility from scratch. I had to accept that I could only do "modified" versions of poses I used to slip into with ease.

A note to flat-bellied yoga teachers: please know that having fat on your belly makes accessing and being in poses different. I recall with embarrassment my first yoga teaching job. I was a therapist working in a women's drug treatment center, had just finished my first teacher training, and was high on the ideas that "Everyone should do yoga!" and "Yoga heals everything!" I convinced the staff to let me teach a weekly yoga class to the clients.

The women in the class showed up with bodies that had experienced trauma, addiction, love, sorrow, violence, sexual objectification, motherhood, youth, aging, and more. Many of these women had fat on their bellies. I taught them a "basic" vinyasa flow. They enjoyed it, but would groan and protest when I would ask them to do forward folds. They would tell me their bellies got in the way. I was so dismissive! I would tell them to bend their knees, to wish love toward their bellies, as though the issue was just psychological. I would smile (patronizingly) about how yoga wasn't about touching your toes, even as I demonstrated forward folding myself in half, flat belly pressed on my thighs.

Ten years later, in my first yoga class post-baby, I almost gasped when I realized that I couldn't forward fold because—my belly was in the way! The fat on my belly felt constricted, smushed, even painful. I struggled to breathe deeply. I felt frustrated because my belly didn't allow me to fold forward deeply enough to feel a satisfying stretch in my hamstrings. Now I understood what those women were telling me, and I felt challenged to love this bigger-bellied body of mine.

Yoga, thankfully, offers endless possibilities for learning to listen to and accommodate our unique bodies. I learned to keep my feet a bit farther apart to make space for my belly. I learned to lift the flesh of my belly with my hands before folding forward to make a bit more space. I learned to lift the flesh of my belly with *uddiyana bandha*, a breathing practice. I learned to flex my feet and open my toes wide to challenge my hamstrings. I learned to incorporate other poses—ones that didn't feed my ego the way my "impressive" *paschimottonasana* used to do. I began to notice myself smiling sometimes mid-practice, just because it had become so much fun. Screw getting my body "back"—I had gotten a "new" body! I found a sense of play and exploration in my practice that I had lost during my years of working to achieve "advanced poses."

## Self-Objectification

As a yoga teacher leading positive body image workshops and especially as a therapist working with people with eating disorders, I often feel as if my body is on display. I feel vulnerable going through the process of gaining and losing weight in pregnancy and new motherhood because my roles mean that my body is often the screen for others' projections and expectations about weight and body image.

When I gain weight while pregnant and nursing what do my clients and students think? Do they think I've just "let myself go?" or that I'm overeating? Does seeing my body change prevent them from trusting the intuitive eating practices I preach? When I teach yoga and my flexibility is not "advanced"—something I have actually cultivated—being less flexible, to prevent injury during these years of pregnancy and nursing with a system full of the hormone relaxin, do students think I don't practice enough?

Each time post-baby, when my daughters reached eighteen months old, my body suddenly and consistently started to lose weight. Probably because my babies started to nurse much less and my hunger subsided, or maybe because that's just when my body knew it didn't need the extra weight to nourish another life. I'm in the process of this weight loss as I write this, and, honestly, contrary to our society's myth that losing weight always feels great—in some ways, as a body image activist and eating disorder therapist, it feels worse.

When I lose weight, I worry—will this trigger my clients? Especially the newest clients, the ones that have only known me post-baby—will they feel betrayed when I'm thinner? Will they wonder if I'm dieting, even though I teach that diets are oppressive and harmful? Will they think that I think thinner is better? Will this make it harder for them to focus on themselves?

In the psychology world, this experience of viewing one's body from the outside is called self-objectification, which is what it sounds like: seeing your body as an object, a product, a decoration. High levels of self-objectification have been linked to everything from poor body image to eating disorders to reduced success in school and work. Women self-objectify more often than men, mostly because we are taught to do so all our lives, and this makes self-objectification a feminist (as well as a power, economic, and racial) issue.

Self-objectification is pronounced in pregnancy and new motherhood. People feel the right to touch, comment on, judge, and categorize new moms. So many mothers I have known as clients and students have described feeling like they were treated as incubators. People ask: "How much weight have you gained?" "Of course you aren't drinking coffee, right?" "Will you be having a natural birth, epidural, breastfeeding, using formula...?" When not judged, mothers are exalted as (read: expected to be) "goddesses," "powerful," "miraculous," and even "superheroes." It becomes hard to share when we feel lost, overwhelmed, bored, resentful, or even just ordinary. It becomes hard for many women not to look at themselves through the eyes of others, to just do their work in the world and feel confident and respected.

Yoga provides a refuge for me from these worries. It offers me a place to let go of the "image" part of body image, and just feel what it is to be in my own body. These days, my practice focuses so much more on the internal experience of each pose than on alignment. I love, for example, focusing in warrior 2 on the energetic spreading sensation I feel from the fingers of one hand to the fingers of the other. In upward bow, I get curious about the strong opening in my chest. Where is it centered? Where are its edges? Where in my body am I at ease alongside this great effort?

## I Am Not My Body

In motherhood, I have now lived twice for a few years in a body that was bigger than I ever could have imagined accepting or loving when I was younger. I have practiced yoga, done good work in the world, and been completely loved by all the same people who loved me before—while being at my highest weights. I've learned that not getting my pre-baby body back is not a bad thing. I am learning this yogic teaching viscerally: I am not my body.

I was me when I was a small baby, I was me in my teenage body, I was me while in a pregnant body, I will be me in an elderly body. I am me at my lower weights, I am me at my higher weights. And my body will keep changing. If I am lucky to live long enough, I will look worse than I do now, at least by conventional standards. I may suffer injury or illness that change my body. I will probably look better than I do now—on that magical day when my kids start letting me sleep in on weekends, for sure. I will feel better in my body than I do now, I will feel worse.

Yoga teaches us about our true nature as pure and unchanging consciousness—even as our embodied form, qualities, thoughts, and experiences shift, transform, and come and go. Our bodies, however, are always changing, and none of us get yesterday's body "back," even if we don't have babies. I use my yoga practice as an opportunity to connect to this teaching and this wisdom, to bring my unchanging self and compassionate awareness to each day's new body.

## My Own Learning about Yoga, Body Image, and Self-Objectification Through Motherhood Has Had Deep Impacts on the Way I Teach Yoga

I have reduced offering alignment cues. I know that sharing alignment with students, while important in terms of safety, is not the most vital thing yoga has to offer. Alignment cues often encourage self-objectification and reduce a sense of empowerment.

I have almost completely stopped doing hands-on adjustments. Even with twenty years of my own practice and more expensive yoga teacher trainings than I can count, I have no idea how a pose should look and feel for the unique individual in front of me. Even if they tell me they have sciatica, and I know what poses are "good" for sciatica, I do not know what that means in their lived experience. I also know that, especially when my body image has been shaky, when a teacher comes over and just moves me into a pose, I immediately think of what I look like and tell myself that my pose (and, at times, my body) is wrong.

If I see someone doing something I believe is dangerous or limiting I now try to use invitational language to encourage them to explore changes in the pose. I ask them to notice: "What happens if you bring shoulders back over hips?" "How does it feel if you bend the knees here a bit?" I hope to make the experience more about developing awareness and kindness to one's self than about the shape of the pose.

I've also worked hard to let go of language that puts poses (and people) in a hierarchy: calling one version a "full expression" or "advanced version" versus a "more basic pose." I want to remind myself and the students in my class that a true advanced pose is one that allows us to be present, steady, and at ease.

## Love Your Body

So, did yoga save my body image yet again? Do I now "love my body" with all the ways it has changed in motherhood? My ego wants to say "of course" and be a really impressive recovery role model or inspiring yoga story. And yes, a lot of the time I really dig what I look like as a mama. I love how my body reminds me of nature: my stretch marks flow into one another like rivers, the flesh at the center of my belly wrinkles like tree bark, my curves roll like hills. But honestly, other times I don't love what I look like—none of my clothes seem right and I wish certain parts of me were bigger or smaller.

This contradiction doesn't bother me much: I believe the mantra "love your body" becomes at best useless and at worst counterproductive if what it really means is "love what your body looks like." A comparison—what would I feel if my husband said loving me was about loving what I look like? (Professional therapist tip: If your partner only loves you because of what you look like, get a new partner!) I'm not that interested anymore in loving what my body looks like if I'm doing it through the gaze I've trained on years of television, billboards, and media-created imagery that values thin, white, young, able-bodied, cis-gendered bodies over most other bodies. If, however, "love your body" means show love to your body, listen to your body, and give unconditional love to your body, then my answer is, unequivocally, yes.

Yoga is the clearest action of loving my body that I know how to take. It feels really good to sit quietly, to move with breath, to turn inside, to explore, practice, learn. My hope, too, is that yoga becomes about loving more than my body. My deepest intention is that my practice enables me to serve in the world: to be a good model for my daughters, showing them that I, and they, are so much more than what we look like, to be one voice against objectification of myself and others, to value freedom and life in all its forms, in all bodies, in all beings.

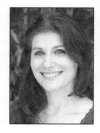

Suzannah Neufeld, MFT, is a psychotherapist, yoga teacher, body image activist, and mother of two living in Berkeley, California. She is a cofounder of Rockridge Wellness Center in Oakland, where she has a private practice focused on supporting people recovering from eating disorders / body image struggles, and around pregnancy / new parenting. Suzannah teaches prenatal and postnatal yoga, leads yoga therapy workshops on making peace with your body, and is currently working on a book on mindfulness in pregnancy and early motherhood for Parallax Press. Learn more at: www.suzannahneufeld.com.

Author photo by Emily Takes Photos.

# NEVER THE PERFECT BODY

## *Dana A. Smith*

In a household of four girls, I was daughter number three: a middle child. While the commonly expressed middle child experience is one of being overlooked, my differences made me glow like neon in the dark. I stood out in every way: inside and out. While my family were social butterflies, having no problem making friends, I preferred the comfort of my room and solitude. My first official job was as a page at the local library and I much preferred burying my nose in a book. Another noticeable difference between me and my sisters was our physical stature. All of my sisters had the voluptuous Smith family gene, which seemed to have skipped right over me.

My family members and close friends of the family would often taunt me about my smaller frame. It seemed very odd to them that I came from the same family yet didn't have the same body type as my sisters. I was divergent by nature, a difference my family just couldn't understand or accept.

Their lighthearted jests began to wear me down. It seemed as if not a day passed without someone making a comment about my body. My comfortable solitude and soft skin morphed into a mobile bomb shelter to nicknames such as "string bean," "bean pole," and other objects void of the dangerous curves so cherished by the African-American community. Even though I knew, and felt, that there was so much more to me than the way my body looked, I could feel the shifts in my ability to feel safe in my own skin. My worth was becoming dangerously entangled with my body, as their fun (at my expense) went on until I jumped ship and headed off to college out of state.

## Enter the Freshman ~~15~~ 20

College was a very different experience: it was the antithesis of my prior home life. In New York, where I was raised, there was always plenty to do and see. Whenever things got too heavy with the teasing, I could easily find someplace to escape. My salvation was a bus or train ride away— away from the fears, the anger, my problems. Or so I thought. Because I didn't know how to stand up for myself, I ran—all the time. I convinced myself this was the best way to "face" my struggles. Now, those luxuries were gone. My small school now was located in the middle of nowhere, where the public transportation system was far less extensive than back home.

As a natural introvert, it took a while to make friends. It didn't take long before loneliness, homesickness, and overall displacement discomfort kicked in with a vengeance. Each day that passed found me more and more withdrawn within some corner of myself, in desperate need of a safe haven. With no chances of finding escape off campus (without a car), I had to find another way to pacify myself. I needed something accessible, quick, and effective. After all, I was sinking deeper into depression like quicksand, and reaching for something stable to keep me above ground. After some searching, I found the answer right under my nose: food.

Food was always a cause for celebration in my house. With my father being a chef and caterer, he had us cooking from a young age. One of my favorite ways to escape when I was younger was baking. Eating soft, sweet treats gave me the same type of feeling as getting on the bus or train; it transported me to a safe place. In my home, the only shortage of sweets was the words I craved to hear about my body. I didn't have a roommate my freshman year of college, so I was fully free to buy and store every kind of sweet and salty treat that delighted me without anyone's observation, judgment, or questioning. I turned to my snacks quite often in the first few months of freshman year. My snacking sessions felt as if I were working through my problems with a trusted friend.

After a while, I noticed my clothes began fitting tighter, and my hips dawned their first set of stretch marks. As strange as it may sound, this was a badge of honor! I was *finally* "filling out" and receiving my birthright of belonging: familial curves. I fantasized about the cessation of teasing and the praises I would receive for physically fitting in. This was way before the time of the camera phone, so I excitedly waited for the holiday break to arrive so I could go home and show off my new body!

## The "F" Word

As I traveled back home, I visualized the warm welcome I would receive. This would be my rite of passage—the moment when I was recognized as a woman among my familial clan. Although that special time had already officially passed some years ago, unceremoniously, I looked forward to being celebrated by the women who meant the most to me. Needless to say, the celebration began and ended where it started—in my head. Once I crossed the threshold into the house I was met with open mouths and a barrage of questions. *What happened to you? Are you pregnant?* Were *you pregnant?* And the most hurtful of all *How did you get so FAT?!*

I couldn't believe it.

As I stood there, grasping for the absentee words to answer my family, my joy shattered into a million pieces. There was true concern in my parents' voices, and I couldn't understand why. As they circled me, looked at my new shape, I felt like a participant being picked apart in one of those god awful makeover shows for their individual style sense.

My brain could not process what was happening. I had never been on the receiving end of the word "fat." It felt cruel. It felt disempowering. It felt as though they were talking about anything other than *me*. I immediately disconnected from my body. Knowing that a negative reaction would be perceived as weakness, I bottled up my feelings and did my best to laugh it off.

But there was nothing funny about it.

## Mirror, Mirror

I retreated to the bathroom and locked myself in. I stripped down to my underwear, something I had done quite often while away at school, and stared at my body. It was different this time. Instead of loving the transformation, I started to view my body through the filter made of the montage of comments about my new physique. My new curves went from being soft and beautiful to something that needed to be changed—immediately.

I fell out of love with my body. I no longer wanted to be that person in the mirror. I didn't know who I *should* be, who I *wanted* to be. My body was too small before and too big now. Was there a happy medium? Could I just do some tweaking and achieve that perfect size? What was that perfect size? Was it realistic to think there was a perfect size that would help me, and others, to fully accept me?

As I stared at myself for what seems like hours I vowed to figure out the answer, no matter what it took.

## Journey to Health

If eating got me into this (body), then not eating would get me out of it. This sounded perfectly logical to me. I had to regain control over my body and even the playing field by controlling how much I ate. Eating was my comfort, so ending the carefree relationship between me and food was a challenge, but I was committed to getting my perfect body.

Each meal I would eat less and less. If anyone noticed I would just comment that I had eaten previously. Finally, I got to the point where I was barely eating anything at all in a given day. Appetite suppressants and energy pills helped immensely. I managed to drop a few pounds before having to return to school.

It was much easier to not eat while at school because I wasn't under any watchful eyes. The weight continued to come off, but other unexpected things started to happen too. I became weak, forgetful, and irritable, and it was starting to affect my work. I didn't like the person I was becoming. It took several months for me to realize that I couldn't go on doing this to my body; it wasn't worth it. I felt so sick at times that I thought I was going to die, and for what—to fit into someone else's unrealistic mold? Even if those someone's were my family, I decided that it was not worth it. I needed out as badly as I needed to breathe. I needed freedom from the entrapment. I had to take ownership. I needed to *nourish* myself: mind, body, and soul. I was desperate for it now. It took almost two years to get into a healthy rhythm with my body. But I made it.

The beginning of my two-year journey felt like hell. There was a lot of mental back and forth, so much so I learned to listen to my thoughts. I was surprised at the amount of negative chatter within. My ego got into the driver seat and challenged me every step of the way, but I kept trying. One day I came across a magazine article that spoke of the power of positive affirmations. At first, I didn't believe that saying positive things would change anything, *especially* if they weren't true. Out of curiosity, I decided to try the daily affirmations as suggested.

I sat down and wrote all of the negative things that I felt about myself. That hurt; then, I changed it to the positive opposite. Each morning, I would look at my body in the mirror and say *I am in perfect health, I am the perfect size for me, I love my body as it is.* As I continued to affirm each morning (even on the days I didn't want to) I felt a shift. The words weren't just words, I started to believe them. And as I did I stopped focusing on my body and started to appreciate it. I learned to ignore comments about my body's fluctuations. As long as I felt good in my skin it didn't matter. Finally, I felt powerful and beautiful in my skin.

## Yoga—My Saving Grace

I found yoga in 2001, while pregnant with my daughter. I was under a lot of stress at the time. I was working a full-time job and doing my best to deal with the physical demands of pregnancy. It was also a highly emotional time, as I lost a dear friend in the 9/11 tragedy. The old feelings of loss of control started to creep back in. My previous method of regaining control through eating, or rather not eating, was not going to work, and I knew it. I needed a new strategy: one that would be safe for me and my baby.

I was introduced to yoga, by a coworker. She knew I was going through stress and shared how yoga helped her to manage her high stress. As she spoke about the long list of benefits, I looked at this woman, tall and thin, and thought she was crazy to think I could do yoga. I was never flexible, and the thought of me putting my leg behind my head—no way! Not one to be rude, I humored her and said that I would consider giving it a try. She gifted me with two yoga VHS tapes—Yoga AM/PM with Rodney Yee and Patricia Walden. The tapes sat atop my television for a few days before I got curious enough to at least watch them.

Just minutes into the tapes I felt something move inside of me. The sound of the instructor's voice was soothing, and I began to follow the breath instruction and a few of the gentler stretches. After I felt calm, relaxed, and at peace. I continued to practice as much as I could and it helped me to remain balanced during the last stages of pregnancy. My practice was limited to my living room, and there were many things I was unable to do, but I still felt wonderful. As the physical pains of pregnancy subsided, my mind went from fear to acceptance of what was. I concentrated on my health and well-being, knowing that this was the most important thing at this time.

When I had my daughter, I knew that I didn't want to pass on my body image insecurities to her. I wanted to give her the support I had needed as a child. I knew that I had to be an example for her, that I couldn't teach her anything that I wasn't actively practicing. I saw my new post-pregnancy body as a work of art. Every line and dimple had a story, a role in the growth and birth of my beautiful daughter. I embraced my body; I was proud of my body. I went through one of the most intense things a woman can go through naturally. I made it through the birthing process and my beautiful body held up. The love and appreciation for my body grew, and I made the promise to myself to always keep it growing.

## YES! Yoga Has Curves

My yoga practice continued to grow over the years. I was stronger and more flexible, and I felt better in my thirties than I did in my twenties. I was blessed with a son in 2011, a full ten years after my daughter's entrance into my life. Those old body image issues were long gone as I joyfully watched my body change shape once again. Yoga was there for me once again to help in the pre- and postnatal process.

As yoga gained popularity over the years with more people beginning to understand its benefits, I started to notice a disturbing trend. The media began promoting the "perfect yoga body." The covers of magazines were full of thin, extremely bendy women who supposedly represented this ideal stature. Gone were beautiful bodies in all shapes, sizes, and hues. Almost every popular yoga outlet promoted this generic and, for most of us, unattainable body structure that represented yoga.

It was discouraging to many bigger-bodied students who wanted to try yoga but knew they could never fit this mold. I was frustrated because this trend was not representative of my relationship with yoga at all. Yoga embraced my body at all sizes. From high-priced clothing to yoga as competition, the true message was being lost. Yoga does not discriminate: it embraces you where you are and people needed to know that. I wanted a way to show the masses that there was more to yoga than what we were seeing. I wanted to create something that would encourage yogis of all sizes, ages, abilities, and races to practice. My offering came about in June 2013—*YES! Yoga Has Curves*. I meditated and prayed that the right people would come forth and help me carry out my mission. And they did. Women from all parts of the world in all beautiful shapes and sizes came to lend their beauty to the project.

If there's one thing I've learned, it's that yoga isn't perfection; it's a practice—one that can take you from the lens of "otherness" into presence. Yoga has a history, it has its mars as do we, but it is a growing, living science embedded in the heart of human awareness, and it will grow with us and in us as we commit to growing within it. The journey of self-love and acceptance *is* yoga.

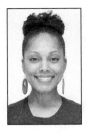

Dana is a certified Yoga Teacher and Trainer, Master Life Coach, and Holistic Health Practitioner specializing in Reiki and Thai Yoga Massage. She believes that yoga is a powerful tool on the path of total wellness and all can practice regardless of size, age, or ability. Visit her at www.spiritualessenceyoga.com

Author photo by Wanakhavi Wakhisi Photography.

# HOW I (DIDN'T) GET A YOGA BODY IN 21 DAYS

## *Roseanne Harvey*

Here's a little secret: although I considered myself to be a body-positivity activist and yoga rabble rouser, there was a piece of me that feared my body, my short curvy strong body, was somehow not "yoga" enough. I decided to do something about it. In November 2013, I willingly took on the challenge of following a quick fix dream body plan created by rock star yoga teacher, Sadie Nardini. The plan was outlined in her then recently released book, *The 21-Day Yoga Body*.

I intended to follow her book for the full three weeks, write about it all on my blog, *It's All Yoga, Baby* (affectionately known as IAYB) and document it on my social media feeds. I was, finally, going to get the yoga body I had secretly desired—while simultaneously deconstructing the whole idea of the yoga body.

As the name suggests, *The 21-Day Yoga Body* was a three-week plan that incorporated a daily yoga asana practice, meal suggestions, lifestyle tips, and affirmations. Each day featured a structured practice that introduced the theme du jour, followed by breakfast, lunch, and dinner menus and a "daily action adventure." The asana practice sequences were detailed in the book and in videos on a website for the book.

"I'm not going to simply review the book," I wrote in my introductory blog post. "No, IAYB is going to do the whole thing. All twenty-one days. I will do everything that Sadie tells me to do."

I started off with a requisite poorly lit "before" photo without makeup or anything. I posed in black leggings and a tank top, barefoot against the backdrop of my cramped apartment/office in Montreal. I looked strong and healthy. I had been practicing yoga regularly for almost eighteen years at this point.

But I have to admit that I didn't mind the idea of feeling a little more fit, fierce, and fabulous. It was November, a traditionally difficult time of the year for me. A few months prior, I had had an abortion, which left me feeling disconnected from my body. Then I'd injured my shoulder, which limited my asana practice (no downward dogs or anything where I had to bear the weight of my body). I had spent a lot of time lying around on bolsters and blankets with ice on various parts of my body.

By this time, I was still a little out of touch with myself, as Sadie would say, on many levels. I needed to shake out some old things and make room for the new.

## Introducing the Woman
## Who Rocked the Yoga Body

Sadie Nardini is a New York City–based "rock star" yoga teacher who created her own unique brand of yoga, Core Strength Vinyasa, and travels around the world teaching it. Her anatomically focused yoga brand is infused with self-help language and the promise of strengthening one's metaphorical "core." She was one of the first professional yoga teachers to harnass the power of YouTube and other social media platforms, and her business savvy catapulted her into the stratosphere of high-earning yoga teachers who attain near celebrity status.

Sadie was also well-known for using body shaming language in the marketing for her workshops and courses. Regular IAYB readers knew that Sadie Nardini and I had butted heads in the past with regard to the abundant use of the phrases "weight loss yoga" and "bikini body" in her marketing copy. In April 2012, I called her out for using "summer body" in her marketing for an online course that promised how to "lose weight and look younger with yoga." I snapped a screen grab of the ad and pasted it in a blog post (which proved worthwhile—after our exchange, Sadie changed the copy in the ad). She responded in the comments section and we had a respectful dialogue. We had interacted on Twitter, and had met in person once at the Omega Institute in New York state.

Still, my perception of Sadie was negative. I fully expected that this project would support this perception. I didn't even consider the possibility that my view of Sadie Nardini, both as a teacher and as a public figure, would shift over the course of these twenty-one days.

## "Yoga Body": Fact or Fiction?

I started off my first blog post by asking: Just what the heck is a "yoga body"?

Luckily, Sadie answered this question in the introduction to her book. "A yoga body is freedom," she wrote, "freedom to be who you know you're meant to be, deep inside. It's 100-proof you, distilled to your essence on all levels, rocking your mind-body-spirit-freakin'-entire-life to a miraculous, turbo-boosted new level. Yeah, that good." [1]

My definition of yoga body (which I consider a culturally loaded term) was a little different. I defined yoga body as "a social construct attributed to practitioners of yoga asana; a body that is most often white, slender, toned, flexible, able, and heterosexual; a body frequently clad in brightly colored spandex and assuming near-impossible arm balance poses." Urban Dictionary offered up yet another definition of yoga body: "the kind of body one develops with years of yoga practice: taller, thin, with legs and buttocks that look like ropes and a bony back and neck." [2]

---

1. Sadie Nardini, *The 21-Day Yoga Body* (New York: Random House, 2014).
2. UrbanDictionary.com, "yoga body." Accessed May 28, 2017. http://www.urbandictionary.com/define.php?term=yoga+body.

The yoga body was something that bloggers and writers had devoted considerable time to discussing, dissecting, and analyzing. Danielle Prohom Olson pointed out on her blog, Body Divine Yoga, "The "yoga body" is a fiction … It is NOT obtained from a regular yoga routine (as many would have you believe)[3]—no , it's obtained at the price of constant work, a Herculean effort to burn calories, and a saintly denial of carbs."

Many critics have said that quest for the "yoga body" is going to be a problem. What could such a body be, other than a slave to a disembodied intention or ideal? Who is "in" the yoga body, moving it like a marionette, and what do they want? What part of us is separate enough from the body that it can reasonably wish to be clothed in a different body?"

It's no surprise that people were thinking about the yoga body, which had become some kind of yoga unicorn, both ubiquitous and difficult to obtain for the average earthbound mortal. The only common factor was that the dominant image of the body that practices yoga is one that excludes a large portion of the population. It sets an example of thinness and privilege that is not experienced by many people. We see these images in the popular media, including celebrity gossip mags (who are quick to report that Miley Cyrus was spotted doing yoga on a California beach, or Hilaria Baldwin busted into a headstand on Fifth Avenue in New York City). But this messaging is replicated in mainstream yoga media, especially in the niche leader, *Yoga Journal*.

I had devoted substantial IAYB coverage to *Yoga Journal*'s body negative snafus, calling out the publication for its homogenous cover models and narrow representation of body types, racial diversity, and age. Over the past few years, the magazine has made considerable efforts to become more positive and inclusive by doing things like hosting conversations at conferences and supporting the work of the Yoga and Body Image Coalition. But it's still limited by the financial and ethical constraints of being a mainstream women's magazine.

---

3. Danielle Olson, "Yoga Body: The Conspiracy" BodyDivineYoga.com, 2013. Accessed August 15, 2017. https://bodydivineyoga.wordpress.com/2012/01/24/yoga-body-the-conspiracy/.

## Getting Out of My Comfort Zone

In my first few social media posts about the project, I reported that I was having a surprising amount of fun following the program. It was great to have the support of the IAYB community, who followed along on my social media accounts via *#21DYB* (shortcode for 21-Day Yoga Body, of course). The likes and comments on the project kept me going.

To my surprise, I was especially enjoying the asana practices. With all this deep core stuff, I did actually feel an inner body transformation happening. I didn't think my external yoga body looked much different (although, I might have been glowing a little more than usual). However, I felt better on the inside.

Anything with the words "yoga" and "body" in the title has the potential to be a body-shaming disaster. I'll hand it to Sadie and say that there was practically no body shaming in the book or her practice videos. The language in both was clear and neutral, with no references to losing weight or "torching calories" during the asana practices. Despite the past body-shaming messaging in her marketing, I discovered that Sadie's teaching style was not at all body negative. She gave options for most poses, invited child's pose in lieu of vinyasa transitions, and didn't pepper her instructions with what your body could become (although "detox!" and "transform!" were frequent).

## A Body that Practices Yoga

In the second week of the program, I posted on the IAYB Facebook page: "Maybe a yoga body is just a body that practices yoga." It got a resounding number of likes and comments such as, "Duh!"

I believe that every body is a yoga body. Even, perhaps, bodies that don't have a regular practice. I believe that every body has the potential to practice yoga, and that if we put our minds to it (not just our body, but our whole being) we are in fact practicing yoga all the time.

But on the other hand, it's not so simple. It was nice to know that there was an enclave of progressive yoga types who believed that the simple basis of a "yoga body" is simply practicing yoga. However, when you do an Internet search for "yoga body," you see that there is a different idea of what that means. Ask one of your coworkers what they think a "yoga body" is. Look up "yoga body" on Pinterest.

As I entered the third week and the *#21DYB* project wound down, I added a new element: taking "awkward selfies" of my body during the asana practice. I zoomed in on my armpit in supported bridge pose, in the blurry background my eyes closed and my face content. I asked my boyfriend to take a rearview photo in cobra pose—he resisted, but I made him take it, and in the final image, my butt looked undeniably lumpy. I posted these pics on Instagram and Facebook, with no editing (aside from a little cropping) and no photoshopping.

I called these parts of my body my "shadow body," the parts that I don't look at, the parts I will to ignore. Cellulite, rolls, lumps, and bumps. I think we all have this "shadow body," even the bikini beach body backbend beauties that we see all over social media. I wanted to challenge the popular notion of yoga selfies. This was 2013, before Buzzfeed compiled lists of body-positive Instagram yoga stars, before figures like self-identified "fat black femme" Jessamyn Stanley were covered in Cosmopolitan, or before the My Real Yoga Body Facebook page existed.

After all, if I was going to embrace the idea of a "yoga body," then shouldn't I acknowledge all of its forms? Beyond the arm balances and lithe muscles? The human body is beautiful, but not from every angle. If a well-rounded yoga practice involves getting to know our shadow side, shouldn't we also get to know our shadow body? If I was going to talk the talk about diversity in yoga's visual culture, I had to be ready to step up with my own body, my own regular, imperfect, healthy, strong "yoga body."

I was speaking to something that Remski had written in his short commentary on the yoga body, which I had posted on my blog: "To me, the real 'yoga body' would be the expression of anyone who gestured at their flesh and said, 'This is really me. All of me. I'm standing right here.'" It was my way of gesturing at my flesh. This was really me, all of me.

## Reclaiming the Yoga Body

I was starting to feel that the "yoga body" is something that needs to be reclaimed (or possibly even claimed; was it ever ours to begin with?). It needs to be reclaimed from Google, reclaimed from marketers, reclaimed from a fragmented culture that has mixed messages and ideas about women's bodies.

At the end of following Sadie Nardini's 21-Day Yoga Body plan I wondered: Am I any closer to understanding the mystique of the "yoga body"? Have I refined and developed my own "yoga body"?

I followed the asana practice quite diligently (missing only two days), made most of the suggested meals, but didn't really make the time for the "daily action adventures." Instead, my action adventures involved opening up a conversation about the "yoga body" and asking some of my favorite yoga writers and thinkers to weigh in. I also documented the project on my social media accounts, and Sadie Nardini responded and followed along, cheering me on my way and answering questions.

I discovered that Sadie has a good sense of humor and is supportive. She seemed to enjoy my progress and was open to feedback. Given the history between us, I got the sense that some IAYB fans were disappointed that I didn't fight with Sadie on Twitter or totally hate the book. That was understandable. It would have admittedly made for a more spicy project if the program had sucked and I'd just complained the whole time. However, I aim to be honest and thoughtful in my writing, and I couldn't pretend to be snarky and hate something that I didn't.

## Before vs. After

It's not a personal transformation program without before and after shots, so in my final blog post I revealed my new yoga body. Here's the thing: it looked pretty much the same as my old yoga body. In fact, it's quite possible that my yoga body may have gotten a little rounder while following the #21DYB plan. I don't weigh myself, so I can't confirm that I actually gained any weight. But I looked more substantial. I had also made the mistake of getting my hair cut and colored during the plan, which some astute readers noted looked a lot like Sadie's own bright red hair with short bangs—it was an unfortunate coincidence, really.

While my external yoga body didn't look that different, I had to admit that my inner body felt different. I felt stronger and more balanced. Having a project to focus on during the dreary month of November kept my spirits up. Doing pretty much the same asana sequence day after day made it easy to note progress in the poses, and I could see where I'd improved and refined.

But no matter how you look at it, any kind of program that promises to transform your body and life isn't preaching acceptance. While I felt good after the daily asana, I noticed an element of striving in myself during the practice. I found myself thinking about what my body could become instead of just being happy with how I was, right then.

This, I think, is the underlying problem with any kind of self-development program. I'm never sure of how to walk the line between accepting who I am, resisting a sort of discouraged complacency (i.e., I'll never be able to change, so why bother?), and desiring to change the things I can change.

My real purpose for doing this program was to unpack the concept of the yoga body. My main takeaway at the conclusion of the project: the yoga body is a myth. If we are diligently, lovingly practicing yoga on a regular basis, we already have a yoga body. Of course, this isn't a major breakthrough. But the whole experience reinforced something that I knew on an intuitive level. The myth was the result of a confluence of cultural factors, attitudes toward the body and fitness trends that have elevated the idea of the yoga body to mythological status.

I also have to admit that following Sadie Nardini's 21-Day Yoga Body plan was a fun and empowering experience. I expanded my asana practice, learned some things about myself, and experimented in the kitchen. After I finished the challenge, I found myself occasionally referring to the book, though I ended up giving it to a friend (a yoga teacher who had difficulty finding time and structure to make her own meals at home).

And my flawed, imperfect yoga body and I went back to my life, to my regular, sporadic practice that fit my lifestyle and schedule, with a few new insights and a few new recipes.

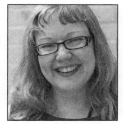

Roseanne Harvey is a writer, yoga teacher, and community organizer in Victoria, BC, Canada. She writes about yoga and culture at *It's All Yoga, Baby*, a widely read blog with a mission to spark investigation into the relationship between yoga, the body, and popular culture. Roseanne looks at the "yoga body" from a feminist perspective, covering yoga and weight loss, body image, size activism, and sexualized advertising and marketing. She is also the coeditor (with Carol Horton) of *21st Century Yoga: Culture, Practice, and Politics*, an anthology of essays by some of the most cutting-edge voices in the North American yoga community.

Author photo by EK Park.

# PRIVILEGE MAKES
# THE WORLD GO ROUND

*Lauren Eckstrom*

My entire life, and yours, cultural and social structures have vigorously ranked beauty. Depending on where you land on this scale, influence and clout may be gained or loss of opportunity may occur. I grew up keenly aware that my appearance would be an advantage, but I was also raised to understand that it could be misused, misinterpreted, and abused. Often, I have felt valued for my appearance over other strong and important qualities such as intelligence, capability, kindness, or work ethic, but I have also recognized the privileges my thin frame and pretty face provided me. I am thin. I have always been thin. I have not always appreciated my body but I have always acknowledged the advantages I've experienced because of it. These same cultural norms exist in the yoga community and beauty or thin privilege play many of the same roles. But yoga brought me to myself and for that I am deeply grateful. Together we have the opportunity to create conscious change in these structures and systems but it will take time, honesty, hard conversations, and a willingness to own our part in how these systems continue to proliferate.

Entering college, I was lost, disconnected, and unhappy. My internal life and my external appearance left me feeling as though I lived in two worlds simultaneously. I longed to feel whole and complete. On the outside, my life was wonderful, but on the inside, I was unsure of who I was or what I wanted out of life, and this tortured me. I was desperate for a connection to myself beyond outer appearance. I yearned for an experience of spirituality and wanted to belong to a community where I could explore these questions safely and openly. During my first few months of college, I learned about the donation-based studio founded by Bryan Kest, Santa Monica Power Yoga. Terrified, I ventured to my first class alone.

Yoga has not been an easy journey. I was never an athlete and, from the beginning, yoga confronted me with a lifetime of programming. Yet I was aware that I needed a physical experience to teach me how to inhabit the body I felt so separated from. Yoga asana forced me to sit with long-held beliefs that I was not strong, flexible, graceful, or physically capable. The practice took everything I believed about my body and turned it upside down. For years it was a love-hate relationship but I always found myself coming back to my mat for connection and solace. It took me five years, a teacher telling me, "You want all the benefits from the practice but you don't want to do the work to get there," and a long break from it before I finally realized I wanted to deepen my practice and study yoga.

## Wah-Wah In My Short Shorts

After a few years of teaching yoga, I felt inspired to share how yoga impacted my life off the mat, helping me create positive and uplifting change in my life and in the lives of others. When I wrote my first article, I submitted to an online community that espoused mindfulness and, of course, yoga. When the article was accepted, I was overjoyed. The chance to connect with students and teachers across the world by sharing stories and to expand community tapped into the reason I first began practicing.

When I submitted my article, I submitted a professional, above the neck, headshot. When the article was published and sent across every social media platform with tens of thousands of followers, I discovered they had replaced my professional headshot with a photo of me in a yoga pose, one I had not offered to them. Their editors had done an online search and replaced my modest headshot with a screenshot from a yoga DVD I had filmed years previous where I was in full extension, wearing only yoga shorts and a bra top. I let my initial surprise wear off because, let's be honest, there are much worse photos of me and I didn't look half bad. I sat down and began to read the comments on the article.

Almost immediately, critical comments started streaming in about my weight, body type, and visible ribs. What I thought was a "mindful" community was filled with harsh comments like "give that girl a sandwich." The entire point of the article was lost and most comments focused on the image appearing at the top. I thought it was my fault—the picture existed somewhere in the online ethers and I knew once I had submitted my article, it was theirs to edit as they wished for the pursuit of mouse clicks. I let the comments and my disappointment go and chose to take the higher path, never engaging with the commentors or responding to the negativity. There were some thoughtful readers who were doing the defending for me, and I was grateful I could gracefully let it go.

The truth is, "give that girl a sandwich" is not hurtful. Making fun of me because I'm thin does not upset me. I know people who have been made fun of or silently judged their entire lives because of body type or physical appearance. To be picked on because I appear "too skinny" in a photo to someone hurts me zero. In fact, due to the grotesque socialization women experience in our culture, I might have even seen it as a good thing in the past. What hurt more than any nasty comment about my weight was being reduced to my appearance, yet again. When we, women, are picked apart body part by body part, no one wins. When we are reduced to our physical appearance for clickbait, we all lose. And that made me mad.

## Learning My Value Extends Deeper than My Body

The site re-posted the article many times over the course of a few months and each time an abundance of comments continued to focus on the image rather than any content actually in the piece. As a result, I finally decided to write a response focusing strictly on that image. I was scared to engage. I was scared to defend what I felt did not require defending, but I felt certain insights were necessary to share in order to address the overt focus on my image rather than my written words. I also wasn't sure if the outlet would accept the response, let alone publish it. Enthusiastically, they agreed and I sat down to write a thoughtful response.

When the article was released, the editors once again inserted changes that gave the piece shock value or increased exposure, shares, follows, and likes, which drives so much of today's media. They altered the title and inserted "exposed ribs" into it. Once again, my body was sensationalized for consumption, but at least somewhat on my own terms.

The image was taken at a time when my physical practice had reached an all-time high. I was stronger than ever, had discovered my true power, and was finally living my *dharma*. Through trial and error, I had learned to listen to my body, to feed it well and without shame or regret. I had a practice I was proud of but was also balanced. The image is a posture of balance but is reflective of an inner balance in which I had stepped beyond labels of "good" and "bad," where, finally, my practice and I were enough.

The most challenging responses to the image always came from women. Women attacking women. Why? How does this help us? Asking critical questions about health and wellness is understandable and important, but vicious attacks and name calling never leads to transformation or paradigm shifts. Men photographed in the same posture are never picked apart for their ribs showing while in full bodily extension.

This whole experience reminded me of a story that was once told to me.

There was once a woman walking on a college campus when she noticed a group of photographers standing nearby on a hill. Curious, she walked over to investigate and noticed two chimpanzees. She learned that one chimpanzee was male and one was female. Neither one had ever seen a chimp of the opposite sex and the scientists were running an experiment to see if they would mate. The male chimp was pulling, tugging, and aggressively lunging after the female. The female finally broke away and found the woman standing in the crowd. The chimp grabbed her by the hand and then led her to the only other female in the crowd and grabbed her by the hand as well. Together, the two women and the female chimp stood hand-in-hand, in solidarity. In the story, the female chimp knew to search out the other women for support.

My question is, can we do the same? Can we hold each other by the hand, stand in solidarity and refuse to be picked apart piece by piece, refuse to play into systems that break us down into body parts?

## And Now the Work Begins

I was able to share my story and connect with others who had faced similar critiques. The article was shared more than 12,000 times. People of all body types responded positively and shared their stories with me. I felt re-inspired and re-connected.

Since the publication of both articles, I have gone on to join the Yoga and Body Image Coalition to help deepen my awareness of yoga and body image. I have become more aware of the issues regarding cultural appropriation in the yoga community, race, and diversity, and I have joined the conversation around privilege, including the ownership of my own. I have partnered with licensed therapists to co-lead body image workshops for women recovering from eating disorders, participated in panels on body image and have re-framed portions of our 200-hour Holistic Yoga Flow teacher training to include awareness of body image and trauma.

I have learned a tremendous amount since my first article was published, but, as a lifelong student, I take ownership of how much more I have to learn. I make mistakes on this path. I have fallen into the expectations that society surrounds my image with. At times, those lessons have been painful and irreversible. But I am learning, I am trying and I am willing to ask the scary, uncomfortable questions that put my race, body type, and privilege on the table as components to consider and take ownership of to help expand my perspective on the students in my room and in the world.

I know I fit the white, thin, female yoga practitioner portrayed in the media, but as a woman, teacher, student, wife, daughter, friend, and stepmother, I advocate for diversity across the board for the health of our world and our youth. And, as someone who fits the current media model, I hope my willingness to learn contributes to greater awareness, helps motivate a dialogue around body image, promotes inclusivity, and encourages change.

I am grateful for my body. I feel strong, capable, and grounded inside of it. Over time, I have learned to wear less makeup and to love what I see reflected back. I released restrictions, removed labels, and granted myself far-reaching permission to listen to my body's needs beyond what society taught me I "should" do as a woman. While all of this is true, it is an ongoing journey, one I work with daily to live holistically, happily, and freely as a woman in the world of yoga.

There are so many wonderful, positive ways to have hard conversations with the hopes of productive actions coming forward and with the hopes of including people rather than excluding or alienating them. Negative social media comments and judgments so often halt the possibilities and are not in alignment with embodied living of yoga philosophy. So, maybe, the invitation can be that those who are passionate about sparking dialogue in these areas work toward owning comparisons and assumptions so that the yoga community doesn't continue to promote the "not good enough" conversation. Unfortunately, comparisons and assumptions only emphasize this "not good enough" program, which I think everyone would like to see transformed into something uplifting. Comparisons and assumptions work against the mission and philosophy of yoga, so let's remember that we are in this practice together, as a community, where our intention is growth, upliftment, and inclusion for all. Let all of our practice rooms be a place where everyone is welcome. Let us have the courage to ask the difficult questions and to know we are safe, supported, and heard.

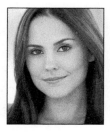

Lauren Eckstrom is a 500-hour E-RYT Yoga Alliance certified instructor and meditation teacher. She leads workshops, retreats, and teacher trainings both locally and internationally. In 2012, Lauren associate produced and was heavily featured in the DVD series *The Ultimate Yogi*, and in 2015, coauthored and published *Holistic Yoga Flow: The Path of Practice*. Website: www.laureneckstromyoga.com

Author photo by Mitch & Brittany Rouse.

# FOCUSING ON ABILITY
# IN DIS-ABILITY OF YOGA

## Elizabeth Wojtowicz

It was a deep craving for oneness and a desire to belong that brought me to yoga. Yes, I wanted to learn how to alleviate and work with my anxiety. More than that, though, I needed an authentic connection to a sacred community and a feeling of mutual support. In short, I wanted to be part of a *sangha*, a community separate from my family. Not only did I crave community I could call my own, I was driven by a deep need for a sense of independence and initiative.

As a very young girl at school, I was incredibly shy—I mean, painfully! I would not speak to anyone and even a "bribe" from my aide wouldn't get me to open my mouth. At home with my family, however, a place where I felt comfortable and safe, I was what one would call a "Chatty Cathy." My extreme shyness with others outside my family, though, was in effect paralyzing me in countless ways. Ultimately, it translated into a lack of self-confidence and led to my increasing disconnection to my familiar surroundings. In fact, I attribute my shyness, lack of self-confidence, and increased disconnection, to that of my disability, cerebral palsy. Cerebral palsy (CP) is a neurological disconnection of the brain to the upper and lower extremities of the body. As such, collectively, my desire for connection, community, and friendship outside my home evaded me and were outside my grasp. Using crutches or a walker to help me get around independently made me feel like I stuck out like a "sore thumb." CP affects my gait (or, the way that I walk), so just by the way that I was walking (deeply side to side, at times crooked), I already looked different, and using mobility aides didn't help me to look less so. I would get a lot of stares from kids and I heard them whisper, all of which exacerbated my shyness. In fact, it wouldn't be until years later where my mama would stare back at the person who was staring at me to make a point. "What? You haven't seen anyone with canes or crutches before?" While it was always said out of love, I disliked the attention those statements drew to me. In fact, her stare downs with others made me want to go deeper into hiding.

## Craving Connection

Often, I would watch my able-bodied family members participate in countless sports; from tennis to soccer to competitions in baton twirling. As I would watch others and their teams compete, rally, and support one another, I was struck with a sense of wonder (and at other times, jealousy). I was often left out, on the sidelines of these activities and, what seemed to me, life in general. As these experiences continued, I grew more and more disconnected from myself and the capabilities I did possess.

I felt small.

I felt like a burden to those around me.

I felt very heavy emotionally.

These are the stories that created deep wounds, wounds I probably would not have examined had it not been for my introduction to yoga years later. At the time, as it was happening to me, I felt extremely unwanted and incredibly incapable.

Surprisingly, even though I was young and lacked experience, somewhere deep down I knew that these experiences would not define me or what I could or could not do forever. Despite my sense of isolation and disconnection and pangs of occasional jealousy and rejection, I knew that these experiences would serve as the catalyst of who I would eventually become, who I am today, and who I am becoming. And that pearl of realization fueled me.

When I was nineteen, I began to understand what cerebral palsy meant for me long-term. CP is a neurological condition that creates disconnection of muscle coordination and movement and it is often a result of a birth trauma. My CP was caused due to premature birth. I was born three and a half months early, weighing in at one pound five ounces. Often being labeled as "one that would ask many questions" (and I still do ... I am VERY curious), my mama shared with me from the beginning that I stopped breathing for a little bit. That lack of oxygen to my brain is what caused my CP. Yes, it was hard in many ways, but after all these years, I see that I was and am blessed with a mild form of CP.

The faith, love, and support from my family is what helped me deepen that connection and realization that although I may not have strong legs like everybody else, I still have a deeper strength and connection to a more magical ability, yoga. I knew it wasn't going to be easy by any means, but I was as ready as I'd ever be to create a newfound connection between my body and physical challenges that I had to work with.

As many of us who are a part of this community know, yoga is about UNITING, creating that unification of mind, body, and spirit, and I wanted to learn how to UNITE all the disconnected parts of Self to create that connection of acceptance to my body—a body that I KNOW was different physically from those around me. I wanted to learn to embrace my disability and the way my body looked and worked, from an integrated, wholehearted perspective. And yoga helps me toward that acceptance, toward that integrated wholehearted perspective of my different physical body. Yes, yoga is physical, no doubt, and I feel much stronger, but yoga for me is more about how we want to show up in the world, through our own hearts with love and when I learn to show up in the world through my heart, with love, it brings about a collaborative connection, that sense of community which then in turn presented me with a new understanding and appreciation for my body.

I was hungry and craving attention and independence, two things that lead back to connection. Connection in turn creates unification, which is what yoga is all about. I believe that many of us (and I include myself in this) do not like to admit that we want attention, especially when having a physical disability. I already was getting a lot of attention for needing more physical help than my younger or older sisters, or anyone else who was able-bodied. Where I believe my craving for connection was quite dominant was when I was in my early twenties.

Imagine hearing things that made you often attribute those words into doubt, blame, and shame. Looking back on that, I would attribute that translation to my negative body image. It was short lived, but at the time of maturity and growth, it established in me a feeling of deep anxiety and shame, which in turn translated into what seemed like craving attention. But the attention that I wanted was connection that would slowly lead to independence, which would lead to me taking the initiative. That deep disconnection of my body and the motivation to understand it, was what brought me closer to that craving for independence and autonomy. For so long growing up, I felt left out of social events, but it wasn't until years later when yoga came into my life that I started to realize that I am independent in many aspects of my life through this powerful practice. Yes, I still am living with Mama and Dad now in my late twenties, and they help me to be in a community with like-minded people, but the moment I slowly get onto my mat (whether in a class or at home), I am claiming my spot. And that is my way toward one (of many) aspects of independence. And for that, I have yoga and this supportive community of teachers and my students to thank for my (growing and evolving) "Independent Initiative."

## Balance in Body

Balance is not only physical but it is also emotional. My life journey with cerebral palsy for twenty-seven years has been what feels like nothing but "finding my balance" (whether it be physically, emotionally, spiritually, energetically) in my body. But what I have come to realize and learn through this practice, is that balance (top to bottom) is what translates through yoga as, harmony. Through the physical challenges of this disability (through many years of physical therapy and occupational therapy), I had to learn how to harmonize the disconnection (and pain) between my brain and my body by paying attention to what my body needed or did not need (and boy, my body KNEW and KNOWS how to communicate what it didn't or doesn't need, let me tell you). And in learning how to balance that and harmonize that, I came to understand that I will have to keep learning to find that balance between my "Independence Initiative" (more so than the "average" able-bodied person might), what I can do on my own with minimal or no help, and what I need help with and how to ask for it. With that understanding comes great acceptance, and with acceptance comes harmony.

Emotionally, I had to come to accept that my body does have to work physically harder to just stand on both feet as evenly as possible (even with crutches) or that I probably won't "do" the Detox Flow Yoga class like the teacher designed and sequenced it. But the beauty that I have slowly come to love about my body, through my yoga practice and teaching, is that the balance that my body expresses (whether it's how to stand, or "Take the Initiative")—that is *my* body's balance and *my* body's way of harmonizing and bringing about—connection. Connecting to that balance in my emotional body is what created that shift from the negative body image that I had due to my anxiety and hunger for connection. It is something that I work on continuously (to the best of my ability and strength), but it is something that I know is in my control and that is a very empowering feeling.

## Acceptance in Ability

Acceptance is challenging in many aspects of our life because life asks us to come to terms with what we have been given or what has been or is presented in front of us and to do the best that we can with what we have. And it took me quite a few years and experience to get to a place of acceptance with the ability that I did have and do have. With this community of like-minded people, I have come to realize that the connection and the feeling of connection is what helped me to accept and appreciate my abilities and capabilities. Yes, I do use crutches and sometimes a tripod walker, but my crutches or my walker do not define me or who I am. I am not my crutches. I am not my walker. I am not my mobility aides. I use them for the simple (but profound) ability to connect in the *sangha*—what in yoga is community. A defining moment in acceptance *toward* my ability and "Independent Initiative" came in November 2015 for a special writing retreat in California. I try to never say never but I *never ever* traveled on my own without Mama or Dad, so when I said, out loud to Mama, "I am going to go to this. Someway, somehow it's gonna happen," I really didn't know *how* it was going to happen, I just knew it *was* going to happen. (This is where being a Jersey Girl Type A personality is gratifying, ha!). But in all seriousness, I felt (and feel) *proud* that I grew up with loving, caring, supportive, hard-working immigrant parents in a state that made you "rough and tough," if you will, because all of those experiences, teachings, and learnings have given me the tenacious, determined spirit that I am proud to possess ... because through the hard work of connection, fund raising, writing, and sharing ... I flew to the Golden State by myself and my faith toward an acceptance in my ability and my independent initiative I did not know was truly possible. And for that, I have my body (and all of its challenges) to thank. This disability is what has given me the *ability* to transform my tribulations into triumphs and my challenges into constructive catalysts for change.

## Tenacious to Teach

It is a blessing and a privilege to be able to share my abilities in a way that may not be "mainstream" but that, in and of itself, is very motivating. Six years ago, when I was inspired to enroll in a 200-hour teacher training course to teach yoga, I really didn't feel scared or intimidated. Ever since I started my yoga practice eight years ago, I never had the intention to teach yoga, but there was something in me that knew that this was something I needed to do for myself. Teaching yoga for five years now has taught me the importance of connecting, of listening, of always learning. For me, on a deeply profound level, there has been (and is) tremendous gratitude in the opportunity to work with and teach people with physical and/or other challenges. Seeing their tremendous, zest for life, for the *breath connecting* to their body (often for the very first time probably in their life), is truly incredible. Playing "Yoga Bingo" as the private yoga class and practice for young girls who learned they have CP, is unlike anything I would have ever imagined. The *joy* in a face when one did butterfly pose or dolphin (despite some obvious challenges) was truly a blessing to be a part of, in their discovery, fun, creativity, and play. Teaching yoga to able-bodied students versus students with physical disabilities, has been (and is) a blessing, an honor, and a privilege. My students teach me so much; whether it's in a private class, a group class, at a studio, or at the Cerebral Palsy of North Jersey Center in Wayne, New Jersey, we are *all* dealing with our own challenges in life; it's just that some are more visible than others. The only thing that makes us different is the attitude with which we approach those challenges.

The practice of yoga and the relationship that is cultivated between our breath and body is what has helped me to learn to cultivate continued positive body image. Being a woman with a disability in the world today in many ways inspires me to be a voice for those who don't believe that they can do it or that they are worth it or that it's okay ... because I have been there. It has brought me great confidence to connect, reach out, speak out toward various issues that are not only happening locally but globally as well, thanks to an *amazing* nonprofit grassroots organization that I am blessed to be a passionate participant of for six years now (and continuing), "Off the Mat Into the World," founded by a dear teacher whom I greatly respect. Through common concern for worldly issues such as undereducated children in Cambodia, the inadequate services for mothers-to-be to give birth in a remote village in Uganda, HIV/AIDS in South Africa, relief and reconstruction of the tsunami aftermath in Haiti, sex trafficking in India, political awareness of the destruction of the Amazon Rainforest in Ecuador, awareness of FGM, and early childhood marriage in Kenya (having passionately participated in awareness building and fund raising with Haiti, India, Ecuador, and Kenya, and ongoing in the near future), I am truly blessed and truly grateful for my OTM "Soul family." I have learned so much about myself; my strengths, my weaknesses, my passions, my curiosities through this beautifully blessed platform of like-minded teachers, healers, inspirations ... Activism for our collective, collaborative consciousness and collaborative connection.

Yes, I have a lot of growing up to do (and as far as I'm concerned, no matter what age we are, we are *always* growing up), but through my teaching, I hope to inspire (and in turn, be inspired) that our challenges, our anxieties, our confusions, our questions, our *curiosities* ... are what make us human, and it is okay to ask, to reach out, because in the end, what we want is a reintegration of connection, which leads to a love bigger than we could have ever imagined. I am honored and I am privileged to teach and practice *with* my challenges, as a way to empower my students (of *all* abilities) through attitude and acceptance.

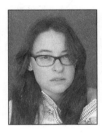

Elizabeth Wojtowicz is a Challenged Yoga Teacher, student, writer, aspiring author, Integrative Nutrition Health Coach, and lover of the beautiful grassroots non-profit "Off the Mat Into the World."
Author photo by Sarit Z Rogers.

# PART 4 MOVING INWARD & UPWARD

- How has our media culture impacted your relationship with your body?
- Describe the dominant portrayal of the "yoga body."
- What would be the personal and cultural effects of not only redefining the "yoga body," but what it means to have a "good body"?
- How does your body image intersect with your race, gender identity, sexual orientation, class, age, or size?
- How do the systems and structures of society operate to privilege some while oppressing others?
- What is one way you can help remedy this?
- What becomes possible when we become at peace with ourselves? How can we support this process for others?
- What does "love your body" mean to you?
- Think of at least two ways you can deepen the meaning attached to this phrase and at least one way you begin a practice of self-acceptance with the goal of unconditional self-love for your entire being.
- Conduct one random act of kindness for yourself today and then one for another person without any expectations about the outcome.

# PART FIVE

## *Igniting Your Inner Yoga Renegade*

On the road to healing and creating change, we must find and cultivate our authentic voice and then vehemently proclaim our truth. It also means we must often re-imagine, re-think, and re-create. Doing so usually results in working against the grain and rebelling against the norm. The stories in this section offer insight, encouragement, and examples of the courage to resist or discard what is harmful or does not serve our highest selves. And we aim to be our best selves so that we may contribute to our collective well-being.

Inspired to share the benefits of yoga, Western yoga pioneer, Judith Lasater, aimed to make yoga accessible to larger audiences by cofounding *Yoga Journal*. She shares the ways in which *Yoga Journal* has contributed to the "yoga body" ideal and how, in realizing she had become part of the "problem," she re-examined her own expectations and judgments.

Cyndi Lee shares her insights on growing older in an ageist society and how this impacted her career teaching yoga as well as her perception of self. After grappling with her conflicted feelings and sense of disappointment, Lee sets out to change the image of what a yoga looks like.

Photographer and activist Sarit Z Rogers chronicles the way in which she was able to overcome her own trauma, shame, and distorted body image to become an agent of change. In a male-dominated industry with an affinity for digital alteration, Rogers represents a challenge to the norm. Rather than accepting the status quo, she utilizes her camera as a mechanism for change.

Rachel Brathen talks candidly on her unexpected and unlikely journey to becoming the "yogalebrity" known as Yoga Girl. In doing so, she serves as an example of how to live authentically and freely despite the heavily filtered social media landscape as well as other's expectations and projections.

Next, Pranidhi Varshney shares how yoga allowed her to move beyond her incessant need to control her body into a state of connection, offering freedom and purpose. As her relationship with her body healed, Varshney was inspired to take action. Not only did she teach yoga as service, she chose to model ways to move beyond conventional definitions of success and create an authentic and empowering space for others in the process.

Similarly, based on an extensive practice of yoga in which *any* body practiced yoga, Zubin Shroff was compelled to create spaces in which everyone felt included and welcomed. In doing so, he completely reimagined the concept of the yoga studio and studio culture then put that vision into action.

Finally, Gail Parker demonstrates the ways in which yoga not only creates awareness but also empowers and emboldens us to unapologetically and courageously walk into the truth. She reminds us that when we love ourselves, we can change the world.

# FINDING REFUGE ON THE YOGA MAT: HOW MODERN PRACTITIONERS NEED TO SAY NO TO OUR CULTURE AND YES TO OURSELVES

*Dr. Judith Hanson Lasater*

All I remember about my first yoga class is the ceilings. That was because we spent a lot of time lying on our backs on our blankets. We would lie down and rest between every pose; the room was dark and the teacher's voice was muted.

I was in the Student YMCA-YWCA across the street from a large university, and free attendance at this class was a "perk" I received as a new employee of the "Y." I was finishing up my thesis for my master's degree and needed a part-time job. I was fortuitously drawn to apply at the "Y" and thus here I was, stretching and breathing with a room full of other university students several evenings a week.

At that time, yoga was an exotic endeavor. There were no special mats or props and certainly not any "yoga clothes" to be found. We began to use small, inexpensive thin rugs for our practice that we had purchased from a chain store full of imported goods. We didn't tell our families we were going to yoga classes. I once did try to tell my family, and I was asked why I wanted to lie on a bed of nails.

There were a number of differences about practicing yoga in those days, and the differences were marked from how practice is now. First, much of the practice was done with eyes closed. We barely noticed the person on the neighboring mat. We were continually instructed to focus inwardly. Thus it was not easy, nor encouraged, to be competitive with others or with ourselves. Competition was not part of the culture of the class. No one seemed to notice what anyone else was wearing. I wore tights and a leotard because I had some stuffed at the back of a drawer in my apartment. These were left over from my dancing days. And that is what my teacher wore, so it seemed appropriate. But, most importantly, there was no standard of how the pose should be performed and certainly no standard or expected way we as women should look while doing yoga. There was literally no body shape standard at all.

After ten months of practice, my husband and wife teacher team moved across the country and asked me to take over the large yoga program. In the innocence of youth, I said "yes" and my yoga journey began in earnest. Now teaching was my only job; two classes every a.m. and two classes every p.m., Monday through Friday. I was living in leotards. And that's when it happened.

I began to fast once a week. Over the next few months, I began to fast a lot and to limit and avoid food. My average-sized body began to drop weight until I was just a few pounds above 100. One of the most interesting things that happened was the amount of compliments I received now for how "skinny" I looked.

I became obsessed with weighing myself twice a day. I developed anorexia without ever hearing the word. I had internalized the belief that my worth and "being skinny" were the same thing. I was so obsessed that I even took a bathroom scale on my honeymoon. Food became my enemy. I avoided social situations where food played a prominent part. I was not nourishing my body with adequate food and, by extension, was not nourishing myself in an emotional or spiritual away. Despite the size label on my jeans or all the compliments I received, I was full of self-loathing.

When I think back to those early days, I see the irony. The very first precept of practicing yoga is <u>not</u> "Thou shall wear a size 2 jeans and be able to practice scorpion pose for the rest of your life." Yoga practice begins with *ahimsa,* "non-harming." How sad that I had not understood that in my early years and, in fact, was harming myself through attachment to my beliefs about how my body should look from the outside. I was not really practicing from a place of deep compassion for myself. I didn't even know what that meant.

## The Beginning of Loving My Body

It was years later when I would begin to learn to focus on reducing my anxiety in general, to look inward to find the inner goodness and inherent wisdom existent in all human beings, even me. As I began to practice "savasana of the soul" through meditation and restorative yoga, I began to feel freer about my body in a healthy way. I stopped reading or even looking at fashion magazines. I tried to go a whole day without looking in a mirror. And when I did, I tried to remember to look myself in the eyes and say out loud "I love you" to myself.

I developed the habit of thanking my body every night before sleep for what it had allowed me to enjoy and accomplish that day. My yoga mat truly became a place of refuge. Just being on it became a refuge. I began to listen to my true hunger and eat when it appeared. My body responded by sleeping better and reshaping itself in a way that was both effortless and comfortable. I felt at home in my skin for the first time since childhood.

Yoga practice, transplanted from the culture of India into the modern West, has been transformed by the culture in which it lives. And this ability to adapt is part of why yoga has stayed alive for thousands of years. Yoga melds with the culture in which it is. Its roots are Indian but its expression is formed by the practitioner's culture. Gradually, yoga began to be accepted in the culture and was "discovered" by athletes and actors and prominent people. Just before this happened, I founded *Yoga Journal* magazine in 1975 with four others, and so I became unwittingly part of sometimes perpetuating an image for the reader to copy.

Our intention when we started *YJ* was to support others in learning about yoga—the poses, the breathing, the meditation, and the philosophy that underscored all these practices. In short, we wanted to make the practice of yoga accessible to a wider audience.

So, one day we met at my house and decided to turn our local newsletter, "The Word," into a magazine. Although none of us knew anything about publishing a magazine, we just moved ahead.

The cultural context of the time had been influenced by the political and cultural upheaval of the late 1960s and early 1970s. More and more people were beginning to find ways to stay physically active, look at different ways of eating, to live in harmony with themselves and the earth. We at the first meeting of *YJ* were part of this process. We were "questioners" and decided to communicate with others like us.

## The Power of Yoga Visuals and Our Self-Worth

Of course magazines are, in large part, a visual art. The writing is important but what draws us to a magazine are the visuals, especially the cover. We on the staff of *YJ* became part of creating and popularizing the images of what a "yoga body" looked like. Our covers were always young women, thinner and thinner through the years. Ads in the magazine became more and more expressive of a specific body type.

We had no intention of creating a certain "body type" or "look" for others to emulate. Rather, in the beginning we were simply influenced by the accepted wisdom about magazine covers: use an attractive woman. So we did.

I remember the first time I read the phrase "yoga workout" and I felt shocked. I wanted to yell out loud to the world, "No! Yoga practice is a work *in*." It is to serve as a pathway into our very self, to help us gradually step away from our thoughts *about* ourselves so we can *be* ourselves. Practicing in a way that is concerned with how we perform the pose and how it looks from the outside is anathema to self-knowledge.

Personally, I realized how much I was unconsciously manipulated in my aesthetic choices by the wider culture. I did *not* realize that in rejecting the cultural standards of beauty, I had simply substituted another one; the Yogic Ideal.

It was then that I realized that I had become part of the problem; I had internalized the normative body image of the yoga world, simply using it to replace my old one. I was unconsciously confusing discipline and control, clinging to the belief that I was healthy because I practiced yoga when actually much of my practice time was spent with an unacknowledged deep repugnance for my body. During my practice I was always telling my body what to do, never listening to what it wanted to do. And so I was desperately attempting to "fix" myself with yoga.

## Food Is Not the Enemy

Even with a cursory perusal of the yoga community in the United States today—the ads, the magazines, the clothes, the attitudes—one comes abruptly face-to-face with rigid attitudes of behavior, beliefs about food, and the strident judging of those in the yoga world who actually dare to eat "the wrong" things.

A perfect example of this was a small gathering I planned for friends at my house; we were all to bring a poem to share after dinner by the fire, either a well-loved poem or an original one. My concept was a "yoga teacher salon" where we could connect outside of our role as yoga teachers.

When I sent out the invitations, I asked for the recipients not only to RSVP, but also to tell me of their food preferences. I received detailed lists of what could not be eaten. But one response was refreshing in its kindness and stimulated an awareness in me about how I thought about food. This particular person wrote: "My friend and I would be happy to come. We normally eat vegetarian, but would humbly accept whatever food you offer."

I certainly would never have said that if I were invited to dinner. I was much too attached to my strict list of what I didn't eat, what I did eat, what time of day I ate it, my ongoing list of "good" and "bad" foods, and especially which foods were "rewards" and which were good for me so therefore I "had" to eat them. The sweet reply that I received opened my eyes to how we take for granted the belief in *withholding as a form of goodness and power.*

It seems to me that we have supposedly taken up yoga to learn to live with open hearts, not just open hamstrings, to become freer in our thinking and acting, to hold all beings as precious and a gift. Even ourselves.

I am not saying that I am not particular about choosing to eat the food that I believe is best for me. Of course I do that on a daily basis. Rather, what I am hoping to raise here is the awareness of our attitude behind the choice. Are we adaptable? Are we present? Are we kind? Sometimes, perhaps, we judge ourselves harshly if we step outside of our food rules. Additionally, I believe that we judge others just as harshly for their food choices, "healthy" or otherwise. Are we aware that we may punish ourselves within our judgments and in other ways when we believe we have been "bad" about food?

These days I am eating in a way that is based on listening to my body, noticing what makes my mouth water, noticing when true hunger arises from my body. Then when I eat, I sit down and just eat. I savor every bite, I bless the people that grew the food, and I stop when I am full, even if there is one bite left on my plate. This process has helped me stop obsessing about food, and, for the first time in my life, I feel free around food.

## Making Ourselves Better

Women particularly tend to easily fall prey to the tyranny of "looking the part of yogini." It was important to me that I really looked the part, both in body and in clothing.

Paradoxically, I wonder if we are using our yoga practice as a way to avoid the state of yoga? Are we using our yoga practice as just another distraction from our own unhappiness, in the same way a child uses a new toy? So our yoga practice begins to serve two unconscious processes: we can use it to feel good about our body and ourselves, and we can almost simultaneously use yoga practice to punish ourselves when we feel we have not lived up to our ideals.

Most importantly, how can we be dedicated practitioners of yoga and simultaneously refuse, with the softest energy, to be captured by our thoughts of judgment about how we should look when we practice? The way we answer this question will not only shape our practice, it will shape our lives.

What is enough? What is enough food? What is enough flexibility? Money? Time? Yoga? Love? I want to practice so that I become enough for *myself first*. One of the most powerful phrases about spiritual practice I ever heard was about how the biggest mistake we make in spiritual practice is holding the belief that we have to be different. But immediately when I hear or read this phrase, my mind says "If we don't practice, nothing changes, but if we try stridently to change, we miss the deep practice of being present with what is."

This mysterious paradox can be understood by clarifying the *intention* with which we practice. If we practice to be different or better, then we practice with aggression and from fear, be they ever so subtle. But if our intention is to turn inward, accept our goodness, live in the miracle that each of us is, we find that strangely we aren't ever different, we never really change.

*In other words, if our intention changes away from control and accomplishment, we find that we grow into ourselves even more, we shine out of ourselves even more, we practice from the inside more and more.* And one day we realize we *have* changed, not from force but from love. Then we have become the yoga, and this not only changes our life, it changes the world around us because others sense it in us.

One way to think of this shift is to consider the *yamas* and *niyamas*, elucidated by Patanjali about 2500 BCE in his *Yoga Sutra*. The *yamas* and the *niyamas* are sometimes called the "ten commandments of yoga." The first *yama* is the most well known and I mentioned it before: *ahimsa*: non-harming. Other *yamas* are such things as telling the truth and refraining from stealing. My favorite of the *niyamas* is *santosha*: contentment.

Usually the *yamas* and the *niyamas* are taught as practices; we are to *do* or *not do* them as is appropriate. But I like to think of the *yamas* and the *niyamas* not as prescriptions but rather as *descriptions*. In other words, a person who is fully integrated acts in ways that are described by such words as nonharming, being content, living without greed, and refusing to use sexuality without compassion and awareness.

If we imagine that the *yamas* and the *niyamas*, which precede Patanjali's introduction of asana, *pranayama* (breathing exercises) and meditation, are descriptions of a person who lives in harmony with him/herself, then our time on the mat or meditation cushion becomes not the creator of those qualities but rather the expression of them. In other words, this is how an integrated person acts: he/she does not harm, does not steal, is not greedy, and so forth.

When we practice in this way, the mat becomes a sacred place, a place where we remember our connection with the whole, whether we define that connection in the language of a mystic physicist or as a mystic sage would, it ultimately makes no difference. Let us no longer get lost in how we look, but settle into who we are. Let us practice with an attitude of commitment but not seriousness and clinging. Let us find enjoyment and celebration on the mat for all our so-called shortcomings and faults right alongside all of the things we like about ourselves.

This is to practice in a way such that we truly cannot harm. To practice in this way is to invite growth instead of forcing from ourselves the "right" things for all the "wrong" reasons.

I used to joke "What are they going to put on my tombstone? We miss her so much because her hamstrings were so loose or her waist was so small?" To practice yoga is to seek health of the deepest sort. Yoga practice may help us become more flexible and to stabilize at a healthy weight and shape. But even more important is to cultivate the health that is defined by the expression of compassion and presence, a healthy state in which empathy for self and others is the default response to all events and all situations.

To become obsessed with how we look and how we appear to others is so human. But it is also human to observe those thoughts and to hold them gently, and with a sense of self-acceptance. Whatever form we express or body we have, we all have our roots in the same "spiritual earth."

So start today. Forgive yourself for everything. Embrace everything. Start anew on your mat in the morning. And remember, we believe that life is strong and love is fragile, but really it is the other way around. Life hangs by a thread and love holds the Universe together. Finding a deep self-acceptance is not easy, but it is the only way home.

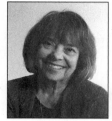

Judith Hanson Lasater, PhD, PT, has taught yoga since 1971 in virtually all states of the United States and on six continents. She is a founder of *Yoga Journal* Magazine, President Emeritus of the California Yoga Teachers Association, an advisor to three National Institute of Health studies on yoga, and the author of eight books.

Author photo by Lizzie Lasater.

# #SELFIE@SIXTY

*Cyndi Lee*

David Bowie died this week. He was only four years older than me and I learned from the *New York Times* that we lived on the same street, so I took it personally. It could have been my door that was knocked on; my time that had come. And it will be one day. In the meantime, I am continuing to grow older, which is not exactly the same as just being older, because it includes the part about growing.

We tend to think of growing as a self-improvement situation; a straight line that leads directly to a better place. This might not be wrong but it might not be right either. From a Buddhist perspective, growing comes under the category of impermanence. That word tends to conjure up images of decay—leaves falling from trees, rotting into the ground, and creating mulch; not our usual idea of a growth scenario. But impermanence can also mean letting go of fixed notions, such as what age is good, what age is bad, where joy and fulfillment are found and lost, and how scary and isolating it is to be older than many, as opposed to younger than most. This letting go creates openings for new ideas and experiences to arise.

Buddhist teachings thus offer a circular perspective on impermanence; all things arise, abide, dissolve, morph into something else, and so the cycle continues. The circle includes things with form and those without form, such as thoughts, ideas, joy, and sorrow. Instead of being stuck in fear, self-judgment, and mourning for that which has passed, these teachings invite us to directly focus on the fullness of impermanence. It's not just loss. It's change and renewal. We start to see this all around us.

The deep realization of impermanence ultimately becomes the seed for appreciation of one's precious human life, as it is right now. This, in turn, creates the motivation to experience life fully, moment by moment. If only we can remember this.

## A Real Yogi

During a recent OM yoga 200-hour teacher training class, I flipped through a copy of my first book, *Yoga Body Buddha Mind*, which was published in 2002. I was looking for a reference picture I could use to demonstrate the energy and alignment of *chaturanga dandasana*. Since that photo shoot happened thirteen years earlier, I couldn't remember if the book included a photo of me doing that pose or if it was demonstrated by one of my yoga friends who was also photographed for the book. But there I was, not only jumping into *chaturanga* but rocking bird of paradise, *dandasana, titibasana,* and a handful of poses I haven't done for several years now.

I noticed right away that I was much thinner than I am now, which is ironic since I remember that the first day of the photo shoot was an "I-feel-fat-day" for me. In preparation for getting my picture taken, I'd gone on a very tight eating regime. No wheat, dairy, or sugar of any kind, not even beets or carrots or corn. Green veggies were okay but no salad unless I skipped the salad dressing. Needless to say wine was out. I had been living on green beans and salmon for weeks.

Then, the night before the shoot, I went out to dinner. Normally this was not a problem because I had learned how to make my diet work in restaurants. But this night I caved a little. I really wanted to eat a friendly, warm meal and not worry about it. I'd been so stressed about all that it took to prepare for this shoot, including writing my very first yoga book! I was ready for a reward and this meal was that. A couple of glasses of red, a salad with dressing, and a yummy fish dish later, I felt satisfied. And also, guilty. I realized that this reward should have happened three days later, after the photo shoot was finished.

Looking back, there was something familiar about this scenario. When I was a dancer, I'd done the same thing before opening nights. After an intense period of hypervigilant dieting and exercising, I would eat a real meal and then feel bad that I hadn't waited until after the show's run was over. Somehow I didn't trust myself to make it over the finish line, or maybe I didn't think I deserved to look "perfect" or maybe I secretly thought I looked fine already. Maybe I was just really hungry. I'm not sure if this was self-sabotage toward my body or my mind/heart. Either way, I felt slightly bloated during the photo shoot and couldn't stop obsessing on the poochy feeling of my belly with each new pose. I didn't yet realize that impermanence meant that however my body felt that day was just happening that day and wasn't really a big deal.

Thirteen years later, I look at those pictures of my slimmer self and envy my own previous body. I can clearly see that I was not fat that day. But what struck me most was not how my body had changed. Over a decade later, I'm okay with that ... mostly.

The thing that caught my eye and tugged at my gut was how much my practice has changed. Since a shoulder issue a few years ago I haven't done *chaturanga*. For the same reason, upward facing dog, (*urdhva mukha svanasana*) got dropped from regular rotation along with binds. I avoid arm balances because they stress the part of my wrist where I once had a cyst. The problem with doing wheel (*urdhva dhanurasana*), began when my dog, Leroy, got diabetes. This led to blinding cataracts that made him afraid to go down the stairs. A zillion times a day my right hand scooped up fourteen pounds of furry love and hauled him up and down two flights of steps. After a few months of this, he got his eyesight back and I ended up with a thumb injury.

Wow, this list depresses me. Even my dog is growing old. My practice used to be a refuge, a laboratory for getting to know myself, my own personal renewable energy source. But the physical obstacles to fulfilling my notion of practice have begun to defeat me. There is a voice in my head that says, "To be a 'real' yogi, you have to practice asana every single day no matter what." Asana practice has always meant plenty of *surya namaskars* with full-on jumps from *chaturanga*; inversions; big backbends, and delicious deep twists with binds. For fun, I might play with *bakasana* into *sirsasana B* straight down into *chaturanga* and through a vinyasa sequence. I was never consistently able to jump from down dog into crow pose and stick the landing, but I wasn't afraid to try it. Now I am. If I get injured, it will take a long time to recover.

Perhaps it's not the practice that is defeating me but rather my fixed notion of how a "real yogi" practices. These days my work on the mat involves all the elements of a yoga class: standing and seated poses, balancing work, twists, backbends and forward folds, as well as inversions, but much of it is supported with blocks and I especially like supine poses. I tend to work within my comfort zone and I no longer practice every single day. Does this mean I am lazy? Or, maybe after all these years I've gotten bored with asana. Sometimes I miss doing a strong, juicy vinyasa practice, but I find that meditation, walking, and biking feel more friendly on my body.

So I find myself in an in-between state, a liminal space of neither wanting to push myself to work harder on the mat nor wanting to quit practicing asana all together. Thirteen years after that photo shoot I do sometimes remember that the law of impermanence applies to me, too. That just like hairdos and skirt lengths, my practice needs to evolve as I age. But sometimes I don't remember that and then I feel semi-guilty for not fulfilling my commitment to yoga.

## My Hair Was on Fire

My first yoga class was in the dance room at Chapman College in 1972. It was the best option for fulfilling my P.E. requirement since I was a disaster at group sports. My yoga teacher gave us asana classes, taught us meditation, led us through *kriyas* including fasting, and even took us on a spiritual camping retreat in Joshua Tree Desert. I wouldn't say that rockets went off when I discovered yoga. It was just a completely natural thing for me to be doing. We practiced in a gentle, easy way with *savasana* in between postures.

When we were assigned to read Yogananda's *Autobiography of a Yogi*, a friend told me she thought the book was a bunch of baloney. "You don't believe that stuff about Indian saints auto-transporting, do you?" It had never occurred to me to question anything in that book. It all made perfect sense to me. Yogananda's story filled me with what I later learned was called, *tapas*, a burning desire to practice yoga. My fire was more drawn to the yoga beyond asanas. I wanted to have a peak experience; preferably an out-of-body moment where I felt intimately connected with all that is. A natural meditator, I spent my late night hours sitting on the roof of my storage-space-turned-apartment, eyes closed, breathing in the rays of the full moon. Being raised in a liberal religious environment, I knew there was something behind the veil of our materialistic life; the samsaric cycle of suffering. There was a natural knowing within me that yoga offered the key to that mystery and I wanted to touch it.

After college I moved to New York City and began a modern dance career that sustained my creativity and social life, but not my pocketbook. So I taught yoga on the side because I was terrible at waitressing, the dancer's typical money gig. When I met my Buddhist guru, Gelek Rimpoche, in the late 1980s, my dances started incorporating Buddhist lessons and my mind turned more in the direction of mindfulness and compassion practices. Dance was losing its grip on me. Bookings and grants were highly competitive and the scene was becoming more about how you looked, who you knew, and the level of your schmoozing skills. I stopped going to dance classes and only went to yoga classes, mostly right around the corner at the original Jivamukti Yoga Center, on Second Avenue between Ninth and Tenth. I also studied at the Iyengar Center and Dharma Mittra's studio on Third Ave.

I had fallen madly in love with vinyasa yoga and practiced it regularly with great passion and total commitment, or, as Buddhists would say, "as if my hair was on fire." The juiciness of vinyasa yoga satisfied my dancer movement jones. The alignment aspect was similar to the precision of ballet training, only better because it is based on safety, rather than on Louis XIV's idea of beauty. Spending so much time on the mat also led me to the discovery that the body is the perfect vehicle for meeting the mind and the exactly right starting point for cultivating mindfulness, awareness, compassion, courage, and joy—everything I was learning about in my dedicated Buddhist studies with Gelek Rimpoche.

Even the teachings on impermanence were starting to make sense as a cyclic thing that was neither good nor bad. But this understanding was mostly conceptual and outside of myself. I didn't yet understand in my bones that I was changing, too. My body, my mind, my abilities, my ambition—none of it was going to freeze at the exact moment of peak excellentness. It was all in play all the time even if I hadn't noticed that yet.

By 1994, I had retired from dancing and was teaching yoga full-time. After several years of schlepping from gyms to studios to privates in apartments all over Manhattan, I opened OM yoga Center on West Fourteenth Street. The studio became a mecca for dancers, actors, and everybody else who was looking for a safe and fun way to keep in shape. The yoga boom was just starting, and I was often interviewed about why yoga was getting to be so popular. I talked about how so many people were at an age where their lives were changing. People in their mid and late forties were seeing their children grow up and move away. Or they were stuck in unsatisfying jobs and their lives felt equally stuck. Yoga offered them a light spiritual touch mixed with a healthy sense of groundedness and clarity.

This was my answer because that was my story. I was forty-four when I opened the studio. The success of OM yoga Center brought me some attention, and soon I was being invited to write for respected yoga and Buddhist magazines.

## Nothing Is Poison

One day I was complaining to my friend, Melvin McLeod, editor-in-chief of the *Shambhala Sun* magazine, about the images used on current yoga publications.

"Melvin, I'm sick of all the yoga cover models being young and thin. I've heard the party line from the publication powers-that-be who say they are presenting aspirational images. But what kind of aspiration is that? 'I aspire to look like that yogini and be able to do that impossible pose and then I will be happy.' No, thanks. We all already have enough 'If only...' scenarios messing us up. Anyway, I know I'm not the only person in the greater yoga community who began practicing in the seventies. We don't want to be told we should aspire to be like someone who is younger than we are."

By this time, I was a regular columnist for several yoga and meditation publications as well as doing feature articles for others, including mainstream magazines that were starting to dabble in yoga-lite pieces for their readers. The articles were usually accompanied by a headshot of me, approximately 1" x 1". I was consulted on who would be a good yoga model for my sequences, because evidently, at the age of 44 +, I was too old to be photographed demonstrating yoga poses.

This was frustrating because I felt like I could do a great job demonstrating the poses I was writing about. Like me, my practice was maturing and my asanas were only getting stronger, more balanced, and clear every day. I didn't think I was unattractive and, in fact, people usually thought I was younger than my age. Not that that mattered to me. I'd already stopped dying my hair, which didn't make me feel old. My gray hair made me feel liberated, empowered, and pretty cool, actually.

My yoga library books were full of photos of older yogis, respected as sages and revered for their experience and dedication to practice. I didn't look at them and see wrinkles or feel sorry for them that they were old. I saw wisdom and contentment and thought, *I'll have what they're having.*

According to Heinrich Zimmer in his great book, *The Philosophies of India*, there are four stages of life in India.[1] First, young people devote themselves to studying with a spiritual teacher in preparation for the next stage, which is that of being a family man or woman. This phase involves raising children and fully engaging in the life of the community. When the children become adults and start running the family business, the parents retreat from societal affairs and return to the forest, entering a spiritual quest to find their true Self. This quest ultimately leads to the fourth stage, when one becomes a *bhiksu*, a wandering beggar, who

---

1. Heinrich Zimmer, *The Philosophies of India* (Bollingen Paperbacks, 1969).

lives fully in spiritual practice with no cares or concerns for the material world.

Perhaps this tradition explains why numerous great Indian yogis have also had more worldly careers. Both Swami Satchidananda and Goenka were businessmen before they became enormously beloved and influential gurus. In the fourth stage of life, these sages become the teachers for the young people in their first stage of life who study yoga as a ground for having a family and worldly livelihood. This is called lineage. The teachers are impermanent but the teachings remain a consistent thread, passing from one generation to the next. Yoga is an ear-to-mouth tradition, and, in fact, the only way you can really learn it is from another teacher; one who has walked the path toward which they are leading you.

And this was the case with me. I was especially inspired by my studies with female American yoga teachers who were senior to me, both in age and experience. Lilias Folan's teaching is elegant and simple, teaching me that a true yogini is kind, straightforward, and full of wonder at any age. Judith Lasater offers a balance of intelligence and joy, reminding us that just because yoga is important doesn't mean we have to get all serious about it. As I was coming into my own as a yoga teacher, I was fortunate to study with these women, who are soulful, smart, gracious, and spend a lot of time on the floor, which keeps them real. And how about Patricia Walden? For her sixtieth birthday, she gave a yoga demonstration of sixty backbends as a gift to her community. That definitely made me say, "I'll have what she's having!"

All of these women have been on the cover of prominent yoga magazines, at various ages in their careers, but now the business of yoga was changing and it seemed that my timing was off. My star was rising but so was my age. No matter how adept her asanas or wise her teachings, a forty-something female yoga teacher was not the media's idea of the up-and-coming face of yoga in America. Part of the spread of mainstream yoga was due to it being moved off the spiritual shelf and redirected to the fitness media space, where it is commonly believed that using images of young, and primarily white, women, successfully amounts to sales. This is not India, after all, but America, and in America being happy about growing old would be a pretty hard sell.

So I was kind of disappointed. As a middle-aged yoga teacher in her second career, I simply fell through the cracks of these changing times. For quite a while, I didn't fully understand that my age was the reason I was being overlooked, because this ageism was unspoken until it wasn't. Finally, one editor plainly said, "You are too old to be the model. But you are very welcome to come to the photo shoot and help the model with her alignment."

They wanted my wisdom, my mind, and my teachings. They even wanted my story about how I let my hair go gray, but they didn't want to see a picture of it. I got the message that my body was not aspirational. And I started to believe it. Over time, I started to feel like these magazines were not for me or people like me. It wasn't that different from when I dropped out of dance. It seemed to be becoming more about how one looked and not about how one felt.

Then Melvin explained something that completely changed my understanding: "Magazines are not in the business of promoting yoga or anybody's yoga career. They are in the business of selling magazines."

Oh. Of course. Even if I didn't necessarily like that answer, it made sense to me. I understood that they have done a lot of research to find out which images magnetize people to buy their magazine and they did not particularly feel a responsibility to promote contemporary feminist culture or provide a corrective to the patriarchal history of the world. They were skewing younger because that sold their product.

I understood this because my yoga studio was also a business. In fact, being a "real" business, as opposed to a nonprofit with tax-exempt church status, was part of my mission statement. I felt that it was valuable to the growth and acceptance of yoga in our culture for OM yoga Center to offer a model that did not separate spirituality from livelihood.

This was another question that arose frequently during the fifteen years that I owned, operated, and taught at OM yoga Center in New York City. Interviewers tried to be provocative by asking, "Isn't it a contradiction to run a business that is about yoga? Aren't yoga and business diametrically opposed?"

My initial outer answer was, "I don't think it makes sense to assume that every business person is spiritually bereft. Or that every person who does yoga is unable to balance a spreadsheet or work in today's marketplace." It seemed like a naive question to me. But, of course, that's why I loved it. It gave me the opportunity to give a little yoga teaching to journalists from the *Wall Street Journal* or *Slate* or CNN.

I explained that yoga is about union, connection, relationship. We manifest this physically in every asana class. Press down to reach up. Reach in two directions to find balance. Feel your breath in your front and back at the same time. Yoga actually cannot be divided. If you have yoga, you have everything and everyone and all that is, throughout all space and time. And that includes business.

My inner answer, the one that I didn't share with journalists, was drawn from the Tantric teachings, which tell us that nothing is poison. Just like chocolate, alcohol, shopping, sex—pick your pleasure—business is not innately bad or good. The vehicle of business can be used for selfish purposes or for compassionate action. Although I knew this and I even had my own business, I was stuck on labeling the yoga industry as "other."

I knew that contemplating interdependence, impermanence, and loving-kindness for self and others was the path to transforming apparent poison into beauty. But it was easier to blame something outside of myself for my feelings of disenfranchisement. As always, practice only works when we remember.

## Selfie@Sixty

Then, one day, some unexpected inspiration arrived on my Facebook doorstep, in the form of a blog piece about how yoga selfies had gotten out of control. My pal, Ramit, sent it to me, accompanied by a question, "Have you read this already or are you actually engaged in life instead?"

Up to that point, I had definitely been more engaged in life than in yoga selfies. I had neither participated in nor followed any Instagram yoga selfie challenges. Frankly, I had mixed feelings when I saw the photos. Handstands in bikinis on the beach at sunset. *Hanumanasana* in front of the Taj Mahal. It was easy to judge this as outsize ego stuff that was inappropriate, touristy, and attention getting. But the truth is that I felt out of it; as if the yoga selfie fad was also not for people like me. Like the magazines, it was more a game for the young and perfect people.

But this day something shifted inside me. As I began to read the blog, I felt the dormant germs of discomfort, self-pity, and rejection starting to wake up. Feeling resentful or left out was my old news; an entrenched thought-habit that had once been a regular and important part of my personal narrative. But since writing my last book, *May I Be Happy: A Memoir of Love, Yoga, and Changing My Mind*, I had applied my meditation practice to this pattern by recognizing it when it arose, gently letting it go, and coming back to now.

It was during the process of writing the memoir that I had finally committed to never hating my body again, no matter what. The book, originally titled "I Hate My Body," was the story of how I learned to be kind to myself as the template for being kind and loving to others.

Near the end of the editing process, I met a very nice man in the airport outside of Tokyo. We bonded because that's what happens when you are in a foreign country during the biggest earthquake in recorded history and you find another person who speaks your language. As people who have survived natural disasters together tend to do, we kept in touch off-and-on for many months. Eventually, we connected again and—flash forward four years—we were living together in central Virginia.

I was happy. He loved me and my body, my gray hair and wrinkles, my squishy bits and my strong bits—he loved it all and so did I. In fact, it had to start with me. The first time we were going to be intimate, naturally I was nervous. At fifty-eight years of age, it takes confidence to literally reveal yourself without embarrassment or apology. So I said to myself, "Okay, Cyndi, you can't write about loving yourself and then be embarrassed about your body. Right now is the moment to finally drop all negativity toward yourself and be free and honest. If he likes me, great, and if he doesn't, okay." So I took a breath and opened to love and joy, and on the day Ramit wrote me, I woke up beside this man, feeling grateful and confident, loving and beloved.

I dissolved that habitual negativity bundle with an exhale, sat up in bed, and took a fresh start. I also included a sense of forgiveness toward myself, understanding that we all have a tendency to blame our discomfort on others.

In this case, the "other" was the yoga media whom I blamed for aging me out and making me feel bad about my physical appearance. But the truth was that I have never liked getting my picture taken because of ego-clinging reasons. I came up in the theater and dance world where photo shoots were big deals, involving much attention to hair and makeup, lots of lighting, and a two-week crash diet. As a professional dancer that diet consisted of cigarettes and diet coke. As a yogi, I got good at the aforementioned regime of no red wine, sugar, wheat, dairy, animal products, chocolate, or salad dressing.

So the thought of a selfie—a picture that shows me as I am right now, today in this moment, without the beauty support system? Well, that gives rise to tiny anxieties that might easily grow into larger self-esteem issues. Best just to avoid photos altogether, right? The article sent by Ramit agreed. It said that contrary to the claim that gorgeous yoga photos inspire others, yoga selfies actually promote this very lack of confidence. Some of us feel defeated and so we don't join in. The blog said this is because the yoga selfies are of skinny minnies, hyper-flexies, and celebri-yogis and not us real people who are curvy or older or less adept in our asanas.

It was encouraging to learn that I was not alone in my feelings. But feelings do nothing but change. Physical feelings, as well as emotions, are completely impermanent. And so are photos. The old days of dance photo shoots where you were happy to get one good picture after two full days of shooting and that picture was the one that would make or break your career—well, that was then and this was now. I suddenly had a new perspective on selfies as perfect, full-blown expressions of the Buddhist teachings on impermanence—this fleeting moment will never happen again, so let's taste it deeply.

What I had labeled as "poison" was simply a vehicle that can be used in any way. Instagram doesn't have a requirement that one be a certain size, shape, color, gender, or anything else. In fact, Instagram is radically inclusive and it was me that had frozen it into something else, based on my own fears and insecurities.

So, I decided to start my own Instagram thirty-day series called Selfie at Sixty. It would show a real yogini at the age of sixty. My husband took my picture every day, so maybe that's not really a selfie situation, but it's okay. The point was that what I felt rejected by—the public arena of yoga that seemed to promote youth and fitness—became the vehicle for me to reconnect to my personal practice.

The Tibetan word for practice is *gom*, which translates as "getting familiar." These thirty days became a way for me to refamiliarize myself with myself and with a new asana practice that works for me now. Some days I felt kind of awesome, but some days I was just tired. And this gave me that path to discover what a sustainable yoga practice was for sixty year old me. It wasn't about doing all the poses I used to do, but what nourished and supported me at this point in my life. It was not about feeling guilty but about applying the yogic directive of svadyaya: self-study through paying attention to what is actually happening, as opposed to what you wish or hope was happening. Seeing things as they are is the heart of Tantric practice. Instead of retreating into our comfort cocoon, we can transform our stuckness into liberation, in the process expanding our comfort zone.

The Selfie at Sixty practice also brought my yoga practice more into my everyday life. My husband and I were on a working road trip for much of the thirty days, half of it relating to his work and half of it to mine. So he took a photo of me in *parighasana* in front of the Washington Monument; doing *parivrtta trikonasana* in high heels on a dock in the Chesapeake Bay, and *viparita karani* on a park bench in red sneakers with my red bike parked next to me.

Then there was the day that we drove four hours for my weekend workshop at Willow St. Yoga in Maryland. I felt stiff and toxic from being in the car for so long but when Brad said it's going to take two trips to get all our stuff in the hotel, I said no way. So I piled briefcase and mat on two suitcases, tossed my purse over my shoulder, grabbed the handles and took a warrior's stance. *Click*, road warrior two became the most popular post of the series.

To my surprise, this daily photo of a mature yogini became a friendly reminder of the preciousness of human life. What can we do with our days and nights? Our every action will impact others, and our own suffering arises when we are too focused on self-importance and caught up in thinking about how we are good or bad.

It's so easy to create our own suffering. And ironically, the very thing that we think is causing our suffering—business, the youth-obsessed publishing industry—can also be the vehicle for our awakening, our honesty, our joy. The Buddhist teachings tell us that all suffering is worthy of compassion and that sharing our story is not selfish but an act of generosity. Turns out that the Selfie at Sixty project not only cheered me up but spread cheer to others via the previously dreaded Instagram. I didn't know what would be gained from this project but I did know what needed to be lost.

Here is the aspiration that naturally arose as I wrote my first Selfie at Sixty blog entry:

"Let me finally release some of this boring vanity and simply open to each day. I want to cultivate more gratitude for my life and the whole, big, beautiful world; for my body and what I can do if I take good care of it. This is not a contest or a challenge. It's a practice. Let's see what practice looks like at sixty years of age."

And that's exactly what happened.

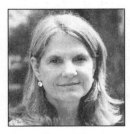

Cyndi Lee is the first female Western yoga teacher to fully integrate yoga asana and Tibetan Buddhism. She is the author of *Yoga Body Buddha Mind* and *May I Be Happy: A Memoir of Love, Yoga, and Changing My Mind.* She is training to be a Zen Chaplain, emphasizing service in areas of women's health and happiness.
Website: www.cyndilee.com
Author photo by Lisa Parks.

# COMBATING WEAPONS
# OF MASS PERFECTION

*Sarit Z Rogers*

I ran from the time I was a teenager, trying with all of my might to create space in a world that felt devoid of love and acceptance. I ran on treadmills and streets showered in the orange glow of sodium vapor light. I spent time in a squat with "friends" whose drug use and drinking was tantamount to my inner voice—out of control and abusive. I didn't think I was worth more; I was told at a young age that I was a mistake. I wanted to be anything but who I was. I wanted to be invisible because I felt invisible. Perfection, self-delusion, and self-hate fueled my internal dialogue and was fed by my anger and shame. Fortunately, I eventually learned to stop and pause. I learned to lean into my shadow and look at it as something that required my compassion. I gave space to my suffering and through that, I discovered I suffered less. I learned to speak kindly to myself and show love to my inner bully. I realized that the desire to be someone or something else was a delusion that kept me away from celebrating the woman I am: strong, resilient, capable, and loving. When I discovered that I could look at ED (my eating disorder) in meditation and say, "ED, I forgive you," I found freedom. When I discovered the wisdom and peace in child's pose or the fierce strength of a revolved warrior, I became liberated on my mat. When I took all of this and applied it to my photography, there was an internal paradigm shift that propelled me to move toward breaking the limiting rules of perfection and creating spaces of inclusion, acceptance, nonjudgment, and love.

When we seek perfection, we subscribe to the message that we have to shift from our authentic selves to meet the expectations of how others would like us to be. Or rather, how the normative culture expects us to be. As a child, I was repeatedly told I wasn't good enough, hearing things like: "You're not normal," "You're fat," "You're a failure," "You were a mistake." The list goes on but the message is the same: I was not what was wanted or expected. I now know that none of what was said was true, but I lived my life believing the lies for more years than I care to count. I starved myself, trying to become invisible; I cut myself, trying to feel; I used drugs and alcohol to medicate myself from the internalized pain and suffering that was overwhelming me.

When I was fifteen, I was photographed and thought I'd try my hand at modeling. At around seventeen, I was photographed in a Downtown Los Angeles Loft in order to create a modeling portfolio. I was told to be "sexy" and "alluring." I was seventeen, what did I really know about looking sexy and alluring? To add to my discomfort, I was naked in a borrowed bathrobe as I "suggestively" leaned forward toward the lens. I felt vulnerable and awkward. I wasn't *in* my body at all. When I left, I didn't feel sexy or empowered. I felt insecure, uncomfortable, worried, and discouraged. When I saw the images, I was shocked to see the perspective of the photographer and how the end result was something that was in direct opposition to how I felt—they looked sexy and alluring, despite my internal experience. This was film, not digital imagery, so the art of photography was different at this time: light and shadow were the paintbrushes and the subject was the canvas. We burned and dodged light onto our images in the darkroom, creating the illusion that artists like Helmut Newton and Herb Ritts made famous.

Shopping my portfolio around, I received a consistent message: "Sweetie, you have the face to go to Paris, but you're too short and your boobs are too big." I was confused (I saw print models like Isabella Rossellini who I thought was stunning and who people told me I

resembled—dark eyes, dark hair, olive skin, ethnic); it made me angry—
what was wrong with being busty and short? I had been fighting to raise
awareness around race and inequality since I was in high school. I wrote
speeches and debated about the horrors of apartheid, yet I also carried
deep shame around my own cultural roots and spent years hiding my
Jewishness as a direct result of experiencing hate speech directed at me.
I never looked like everyone else, and the rejection from the modeling
industry slammed the nail in the coffin: I really wasn't enough. This
gave me something to protest and fight about.

I experienced my disappointment by internalizing it. The message
I received was an echo of the negative messaging I heard in my childhood: "You're not normal," "You're a failure." Having it confirmed by
an industry that perpetuates perfection and competition and yet defines our pop cultural norms felt like the ultimate slam. I starved myself
further—I cut, I burned, I measured, I smoked, I drank, I screamed, I
fought.

## I Need Help

What I needed was help from my internalized trauma, abandonment,
anxiety, depression, and self-harming and addictive behavior. In high
school, I had sought out therapy that was provided by my school. I
asked for help at sixteen. I knew I was in trouble. At seventeen, I got
sober through a program called Palmer Drug Abuse Program (PDAP),
where I went to meetings. I broke up with my heroin-addicted, violent
boyfriend and got my first job in the film industry, where I worked as a
costumer for almost a decade. I had an insider's view of this industry I
was so angry at. Things were different with moving cameras though,
all of I sudden I found myself roller-skating in a bikini for some crazy
B-movie. Turns out I was miserable in front of the camera, still battling
the violent internal dialogue of "you're not really pretty enough or tall
enough or thin enough."

As a youth, I played with sun salutations on the Santa Monica beach,
saluting the sun at sunset. I remember "knees, chest, chin" in the sand,
feeling my feet caress the ground beneath me, and the ocean breeze
on my skin. I remember feeling whole in those moments, however

brief they were. I wish I had continued to practice, but I didn't. I didn't come back to yoga until I got pregnant with my son. My body remembered the asanas, but it took time for me to get my mind to let go. I still avoided public classes because I felt like I didn't "fit in," I wasn't flexible enough or thin enough. I used tapes until they wore out. But I was lacking in the community that yoga represented. It took years for me to come to my mat in public, but when I did, that is when my healing began to take place. I had a profound shift in my self-perception. It was in those communal spaces where I felt supported by community and able to lean into the unwinding of my heart. I learned to cry without judgment, fall without judgment, laugh with abandon, and I remembered how to dance.

## Growing into My Activist Feet

I was five when I first saw an image come to life in the dark, chemical-laden space of the darkroom. I remember the sense of fascination I felt as it emerged. We had a darkroom in our home and it quickly became a space of solitude, curiosity, and emotional safety. I learned that once inside, there was a peaceful, methodical practice of technical and artistic savvy. This isn't where my activist brain was ignited, however.

I became increasingly disturbed by the injustices I saw in the world at large. I spoke out loudly, in the voice of someone who had just discovered how unjust the world was—there was self-righteous anger, which I later discovered is a legitimate part of an activist's growth process! I then focused my lens on my immediate surroundings, becoming more and more aware of the injustices close to home. Anti-Semitism was already something I faced. "Dirty Jew," "kike," et cetera, crashed upon my heart since my youth, coupled with the issues around my name and the pervasive question, "What are you?" The rage stayed with me for years, but it wasn't particularly useful in terms of effecting change of any kind. I just looked like an asshole, if I'm honest.

As I "grew up," so did my activism. Putting myself through Santa Monica College's photography program, I found my visual voice through creating conceptual imagery and in capturing realistic depictions of musicians by honoring their humanity. I photographed my first series on medium format film with my beloved Hasselblad and printed everything by hand. It was partly my desire to control the outcome of the image, maintaining its authenticity, and also part and parcel to my internal discovery of my own creative voice.

I repeatedly pushed the envelope when it came to "embracing" Photoshop and Lightroom. I remember sitting in my Advanced Photoshop class bereft at the idea of "fixing" someone's face because it "didn't look right." At one point, I was told I wouldn't succeed if I didn't embrace Photoshop or the digital world like everyone else. Clearly, that rubbish didn't stop me from pushing forward.

The truth is, I have embraced Photoshop in some ways while tossing its pervasively harmful characteristics to the side. Photography is a lie. Photographers are trained to play with light to create shadows and highlights that celebrate our fine features, while hiding our "undesirable" features. Reality is important to me, and I reveled in the masters before me who celebrated reality and frowned upon such things as even cropping images to make them "look better." I'm talking about the greats like Ansel Adams, Imogen Cunningham, John Paul Edwards, Sonya Noskowiak, Henry Swift, Willard Van Dyke, and Edward Weston, who founded the F-64 group that demanded reality and truth in photography. They believed that "photography, as an art form, must develop along lines defined by the actualities and limitations of the photographic medium." This is a foundational piece for me in my personal work and my published work. I do crop, but I make every effort to keep it real and authentic and accessible.

I hear fashion photographers and retouchers state that hairlines need to be lowered; I find that silly and absurd. What's wrong with the beautiful hairline you're born with? I don't want to be part of the problem that's created when we shift our outsides to satisfy a marketing team or pop culture media paradigm. I seek to guide people toward self-acceptance and self-love. That's no easy feat—we are all subject to the blasts of perfection through social media.

## Visual Conversation and Collaboration

I view photography as a visual conversation. As a writer, I knew I could communicate well with language, but as a photographer, communicating in a visual albeit two-dimensional way was different. I started to intuit fear and nervousness in my photographic subjects as soon as they stepped in front of my camera; I often saw sadness in the moments when I was purportedly not looking. I realized there was a divide—a bridge of communication that not only needed to be built but also needed to be nurtured from the ground up. The inherent judgment and objectification seen in photography had to be squashed. A shift needed to happen.

My camera is an extension of me, but to illustrate that, I have to lay a foundation of trust and safety before I photograph someone. Creating trust and safety and cultivating awareness is another way for me to lean into my yoga practice. Often times, I find myself putting my camera down entirely. Each person's needs are unique to them, and I have found that my ability to pause and attune is what allows me to sense what is happening underneath the surface. In order to cultivate trust, it is vital for me to recognize each person's humanity and remove judgment. I see you. I hear you. I respect you. Without that, there is no trust, there is no connection, and there is no photograph, and there is no yoga.

Yoga is where the rubber meets the road for me. It is where I can discover the felt sense—the embodiment of our sensory, energetic, and emotional landscape, by using my breath to bring awareness to the connection of my mind and body. Yoga gives me the freedom to show up just as I am: short arms, large breasts, and strong legs, tired or awake. I honor my body on my mat: what do I *need*, not what should I *look like*. As a result, this practice flows into all aspects of my life. Photography is an extension of my practice, as is parenting or being a friend or simply being human. What doesn't fit anymore is the false idea of perfection. In the Oxford Dictionary, *perfection* is defined as "the condition, state, or quality of being free or as free as possible from all flaws or defects," or a "person or thing perceived as the embodiment of perfection." [1] But I

1. Oxford English Dictionary, 2nd ed., s.v. "perfection."

ask you, how is this possible? Don't we all contain flaws? Don't we all contain imperfections? And what if those flaws really aren't something to be changed? For example, what if my short arms are left alone in an image instead of being stretched to look elegant and long? What if I stop pushing my arms to stretch beyond their capacity and use a strap to lengthen them in a yoga pose? If we don't find a way to accommodate ourselves in our practice, we aren't doing yoga; we aren't meeting ourselves where we are. Instead, we are reaching for where we are not. Likewise, in meditation, finding safety on the cushion is just as pertinent. If closing our eyes places us in the trap of a trauma flashback, we have to allow ourselves the freedom and the grace to open our eyes. There is simply not a perfect way to do a pose or to sit. Perfection is a delusion we are trying to seize to increase our sense of pleasure and satisfy our greed. To shift this paradigm of desire for the impossible means accepting where we are, as we are.

My photographic process is imbued with the dharmic practices, which lead me to create by the dharmic truths of *metta* (loving-kindness), *sangha* (community), *muditta* (sympathetic joy), *karuna* (compassion), and *upekkha* (equanimity). I need to be grounded in my own truth and awareness if I want someone to be grounded in theirs. The camera is merely a tool to capture this awareness in a moment. Henri Cartier-Bresson, the French photographer who birthed street photography, was also the one who coined the phrase and spoke about certainty of "the decisive moment" in photography. He said, "There is a moment where everything comes together in unison." [2] He's right; in each moment, there is the release of the breath, the dropping of the shoulders, the wave crashing at the right moment, the light caressing a cheek, or perhaps laughter. The moments are fast and changing. The practice is in rolling with that change.

## Change Is Necessary

When I started photographing yogis, I was stunned to see the homogenized imagery that prevailed in all of the mainstream magazines. Here

2. Henri Cartier Bresson, *Henri Cartier Bresson: The Decisive Moment* (1952).

we had an East Indian, dharmic practice with the face of whiteness, youth, and hyper-flexibility as its poster child. In an effort to bring this practice to the West, the media was effectively whitewashing and "perfecting" the asana—commodifying the spiritual to make it digestible for the masses. Not only was this in direct contradiction to the practice itself, it is also fundamentally inaccessible. And despite being of a relatively normative size, I again didn't see myself in these images. I was once again reminded that I wasn't the desired image or "perfect" size. This is similar to my experiences from my youth, where I knew I had to look like some unattainable image to be desirable. Again, I saw height I didn't have, a spine that moved in a way that mine didn't, legs that were long and thin, and hair that was as blond as the skin was fair. I wasn't seeing people of color, I wasn't seeing rounder bodies, or "average" bodies, I wasn't seeing differently abled bodies, or old bodies. I essentially wasn't seeing the diverse range of reality and, in that way, it didn't feel authentic.

I was seeing a false representation of something that is supposed to sell you and me the idea of getting "spiritually fit" through the mindful lift of your back leg to your head. The problem with that model of "perfection" is when we practice yoga and meditation and begin the process of leaning in, and when we meditate on our cushion or our mat, we are going to face our very real shadows—what I call "the time to pull on the mud boots and start slogging through." Even though things get sticky and muddy, it's what this practice is about. Those blasted shadows provide the cracks for the light to get in. Shadows are in the art we create, in that we are forced to sit with the uncomfortable or perhaps some past trauma or our self-doubt. Photography tends to bring this out because it forces us to be vulnerable. Since I am the one in control of the ultimate image, I choose to lean in with the person I'm photographing instead of plainly directing. That, in and of itself, lends itself to authenticity. This shadow work is essential; it is a very necessary part of creating art. It's what leaning in and letting go is about.

Without the shadow, there is no light, and without light, there is no shadow.

I, too, am subject to the media barrage of self-hate and false perceptions. I see images of myself that don't resemble me at all. I can see three reflections in a day, all from different mirrors, all looking back at me differently. Reality has to be what we make it. It has to be how we feel, not how we look. How we look will change. Our hair will fall grey, our waists may widen, our breasts and asses may eventually sag or broaden. But it's our hearts—the resilient muscle that reviles negative reflection. The resilience and rhythmic beat pulls us back to ourselves, back to our truth, back to reality. Back to why we practice, why we lean in, why we take the risk to create art and capture moments in time and place.

When I am photographing someone or something, I am responsible. I hold in my hand a tool that captures moments in time; it captures joy and sadness, love and loss, depression and freedom, stillness and motion. But it is a long, phallic instrument directed toward my subject, placing them under observation and objectification. While I can't stop that reality, I decide how I use that tool. I can shift it and lower the phallis to make the process equal and accessible. I can place my camera beneath our eyes; I can hand it to my collaborator and allow them to turn it on me. Here, the subject becomes a collaborator. The photographic process becomes a partnership. It's tantamount to the partnership we cultivate with our breath on our mats or on our cushions. When I'm holding my breath, I can't let go, I can't lean in. When I fight my breath or push against it in a pose, how deep can I really go? When I take this dharmic practice and pair it with my camera, I allow myself to become a part of the healing process of leaning in and effecting change instead being part of the damaging problem of sameness.

My camera is not a weapon of mass perfection. Instead it is a conduit of change, a tool I use to make an offering and to find redemption from the lies we are forced to swallow when we open our media. Instead of using my camera to create something that forces beauty upon us, I use it as a tool to celebrate and encompass the beauty that already exists in each individual or group that I have the honor to photograph. I want to see people grow taller because they *feel* taller on the inside, not because I digitally elongated their legs in a computer program. I want to see those smile lines, because goddamn it, you earned them! You laughed and cried and expressed emotion to earn those beauties! This doesn't mean I'm the anti-Photoshop, it just means that I have learned to use it for good instead of evil.

We are all "good enough" to be photographed. No, you don't have to touch your toes to your head with a hyper real background to be beautiful. You simply are beautiful. I named my camera Artemis, goddess of the hunt and protector of women. I named my camera Artemis because I want to honor and protect our truth and our inner warrior that thrives on love and connection, respect, and being seen wholly and without judgment. She is not a weapon of mass perfection. She is a channel of love and respect.

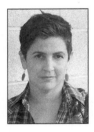

**Sarit Z Rogers** is a Los Angeles–based photographer, writer, activist, and yogini. She is the founder of the LoveMore Movement and can be found at LoveMoreMovement.com and SaritPhotography.com.

Author photo by Joseph Rogers III / Sarit Photography.

# YOGA GIRL: LIVING AUTHENTICALLY IN THE SOCIAL MEDIA WORLD, AN INTERVIEW WITH RACHEL BRATHEN

*Melanie Klein*

**MK:** Rachel, I am so thrilled to include your voice in this book. Given your incredible reach and life in the public eye as an accidental "yoga celebrity" or "yogalebrity" …

**RB:** Yes, very accidental.

**MK:** Right! And given that unique and influential place in yoga culture, you experience a lot of benefits, but you're also the object of scrutiny as more and more people challenge the intersection of the yogalebrity and consumer culture with yoga imagery. Yours is a compelling and unusual story.

**RB:** Yeah, it's an important conversation to have.

**MK:** Well, I'd love to begin by having you describe your body image story and a brief history of your relationship with your body.

RB: I was born and raised in Sweden. Funny enough, I was there just a couple months ago, and while I was helping cleaning out a garage, I found an old diary of mine that I kept as a young teenager, roughly ages thirteen to fifteen years old. Reading it was eye-opening because what I remember and what I wrote didn't mesh. I thought I liked my body at the time, but reading my diary I found numbers at the top of every page. It took me a couple minutes of reading before I actually remembered what I was writing about—the numbers in the top corner of every single page was my recorded weight and a little plus and/or minus sign. Every single day. I guess this is something that I've repressed [laughter] or it was something so normal that I don't recall it. But every day I would step on the scale and, even though I was very tall and thin growing up, if I gained a gram, I would put like a plus on the end and that would mean it was a bad day. That meant that I would have to eat less the next day.

MK: Unfortunately, that's a familiar scenario. In many ways, it's what "girls do."

RB: Right, and it's particularly striking to me now because I was never overweight growing up. Plus, because I was competing in track and field as well as doing gymnastics, I was always working out and was quite fit in the stereotypical sense.

MK: Yeah, a lot of people assume that a negative body image or body image issues only impact people who are overweight or not conventionally attractive. In my work as a body image advocate and media literacy advocate, I've found time and time again that that is simply not true.

RB: Exactly, even though I was genetically very tall and thin as well as traditionally fit from playing sports, I still had this idea that I wasn't enough. I look back at photos and I'm surprised when I discover how I felt about my body. So that feeling of insecurity has always been there.

MK: We grow up with so many influences on our body image or perception of self. Are you able to trace this feeling back?

RB: I grew up around adult women and role models in my life who were dealing with their own body image issues. I didn't fully learn about the depth of their struggles until later, but I'm certain that their behaviors, habits, and relationships with food and their bodies impacted me more than I was conscious of at the time. When I began to realize that the biggest role model in my life—my mom—had been struggling with an eating disorder, it made absolute sense, and a lot of things fell into place.

MK: That's common, that toxic relationship with food and self as an intergenerational inheritance. Have you ever spoken to her of it?

RB: We've spoken about it a lot now that I am pregnant with a daughter. She told me she remembers being nine months pregnant and putting her fingers down her throat to throw up. It's so intense to think about—she was pregnant with me!

MK: You said that a lot of things fell into place for you after her bulimia was revealed to you. What sorts of things?

RB: I remember a lot of little comments. I'm quite tall and my mother is a tiny person. In fact, I'm almost twice the size of my mom! I remember standing next to her in the mirror and she'd say, "Isn't it fascinating that you're only fifteen and already bigger than me?"

MK: That sounds familiar! "Big" was not code for pretty, attractive, desirable, or acceptable. "Big" was bad—a source of shame.

RB: Exactly. I never developed a clinical eating disorder and I feel like I was able to get a grasp of my own worth fairly early in life, but those negative feelings about myself go way back in my life and certainly had an impact. It's funny, though, when I think back on my mid to late teen years, I have a completely different memory of myself.

MK: What do those memories of teen Rachel look like?

RB: I was a rough teenager, incredibly cocky and confident (or so I thought I was). I had this idea that I was the best and on top of the world, no problems at all. Looking back at what I was writing when I was alone contradicts that image. Even so, while it was common for many of my friends and peers to talk down to themselves, I was never one to say, "I need to work out" or "I can't believe I ate that." Instead, I would object to that negativity with statements like, "Eat whatever you want, who gives a shit!" I was all about portraying myself as strong, one who didn't obsess over these things and someone who loved myself as is. But, behind closed doors, there was another story that I just wasn't talking about (or really consciously aware of myself).

MK: It sounds like you were rebelling against the insecurities you'd inherited. Often, though, this doesn't happen until much later in life. But here you were, a teen rejecting the norm and, unknowingly, serving as a role model to an alternate experience for your friends and peers, one that doesn't bow down to the scale or the beauty standard of the day.

RB: I wanted to stand out and be different. I wanted to go my own way and not become defined by the same warped image my mother grew up with. It may have been unconscious, but I understood that her negative comments were always a reflection back to her and, sadly, how she felt about herself. I wanted to rebel against this idea that it's natural or normal to not like yourself and who you are. Yoga was a big part of that journey.

MK: When and how did yoga come into the picture?

RB: I was seventeen or eighteen and, again, it came from my mom. I was on a destructive path, a truly horrible time that involved a lot of smoking, drinking, and some drug use. It was all symptomatic of my unhappiness with my life and who I was becoming. My mother went on a meditation retreat and, later, she booked a one-week retreat for me, bought me a train ticket, and said, "I had an amazing experience and I think you should do it, too."

MK: So you jumped in and…

RB: It changed my whole life 100 percent. It was the beginning of finding yoga and a whole new life.

MK: Given that it was a one-week retreat, your first experience was concentrated and intensive.

RB: Yeah, it was super intense. Honestly, that was probably the only way it would have happened for me. I needed to go all in. I mean, I didn't know anyone who meditated and I was terrified. In fact, I almost turned around and took the train home on the first day.

MK: But you stayed. And what did you experience?

RB: It was an Osho style meditation, dynamic meditations that involved movement and combined with a Vipassana style of sitting. The idea is to move and get all the crazy out before you find silence. I think for a seventeen- or eighteen-year-old, that approach was perfect. In addition to movement and sitting, there was a lot of sharing, talking, and the releasing of emotions. This holistic approach that precedes the actual moments of silence allowed me to get to a place I don't think I would have reached if I had been expected to sit down and meditate seven hours a day.

MK: I think it's fascinating and incredibly beautiful that your mother was the root of so many of your struggles related to self-worth, yet she also introduced you to the tools that have served you (and continue you to serve you).

RB: See, that's our whole path—it's a struggle and a lesson [laughter].

MK: And how did this new practice impact you when you were first introduced?

RB: One of the first things I realized was that I wasn't happy. Despite having a boyfriend and lots of friends, I didn't know what I wanted to do with my life. For the first time in my life, I found a quiet space in my mind and realized that, not only was I not happy, I wasn't in charge of my own life. I'd just gone along with everyone and everything around me, never truly discovering what made me happy. Up until then, I'd never questioned anything before. This was an empowering moment. Upon finding meditation, it became clear that I needed time and space to find my own path. Had it not been for those moments of silence, I don't know if I would have ever realized that I had the ability to choose for myself.

MK: And how did this new practice integrate with and/or change your life, as you said, when you returned home?

RB: Well, I come from a complicated family and have a troubled past. I'd been a part of a lot of destructive relationship patterns and, upon returning home, I stepped away from it for the first time. That was the biggest thing I could do in choosing for myself. In doing so, it was one of the first steps in becoming my own person. My newfound meditation practice was incredibly personal to me and, even though my mom introduced me to it, I didn't share it with anyone. Whereas my mom was older when she discovered this practice, I was young enough that I could make dramatic changes and reshape my life. And I decided that I wanted to find the path to happiness, not a road of constant struggle or drama. I would have never gotten there had it not been for the meditation, which has always been more important than the physical practice for me.

**MK:** Well, learning about your background makes so many of the puzzle pieces fall into place. Looking at the things you've shared (and how you've shared them) over the years, this choice to follow the path to happiness and rewrite the dysfunctional narrative in your life becomes evident. And I think that's a large part of your appeal to the millions who follow you. You're open, honest, vulnerable, and, in the midst of it all, you seek the light, the joy, and that way into happiness.

With that said, the first time I remember seeing you was on *Elephant Journal* over five years ago on a SUP (stand up paddleboard) yoga video (which blew me away, by the way). So, you did develop a physical practice, and many online know you for your physical practice. When and how did that develop?

**RB:** Shortly after my first retreat, I went back for another ten-day retreat. I walked into the *shala* early one morning and saw a woman on her yoga mat. I'd never seen anyone practice physical yoga. She was so focused and looked graceful and comfortable in her body. It blew my mind. After I returned home, I took a leap and moved to Costa Rica. I found a studio there and started taking classes here and there. I also got a book on yoga asana, but I never had a proper teacher. I also didn't have the same "aha" moment many students get in a yoga class (or the "aha" I got in meditation). Because of scoliosis and back pain, I was actually very nervous to start a physical yoga practice. Those first years, I mostly explored on my own—what worked, what didn't work. The first two years were very slow and involved lots of restorative work, the use of props and was very Iyengar-based. Despite my experiences with sports growing up, I had never done anything like this before. Why does my body feel the way it does? Why do I have this pain? Where does it come from? How can I heal it? There was no stand-up paddleboard yoga. There were no handstands, none of that.

MK: Given how many people are introduced to the idea of yoga through studio culture or the representation of yoga practice and "yoga bodies" in the media these days, your discovery was very unique and personal. I think that is incredibly unique and rare, someone with your reach that doesn't tag every single post with corporate tags and endorsements.

RB: I know a lot of people find their way to yoga practice through my social media accounts or take their first class because of something they see online. That may feel strange to me because my journey was so different (and much more private), but it's great that it's accessible in a way that people can find inspiration easily.

MK: Your content has remained raw and feels incredibly authentic, especially without the corporate tags.

RB: Thank you, I fight very hard for it to stay that way. In the beginning, though, I actually thought "Yoga Girl" was so stupid, I don't even remember why I chose that name. It was a personal account and a spur of the moment decision to name it that. Whereas now, I can see that the name was an important part of building community and it felt accessible because it wasn't a slick, branded identity. I struggle with the balance between the commercial world and what yoga is everyday. I realize you don't need to go down that road, actually.

MK: I appreciate you saying that. One of the biggest things in my work has been challenging the dominant imagery in media culture that is so incredibly one-dimensional and not representative of the mass population. And part of that task is creating new imagery through the Yoga and Body Image Coalition, sharing these stories, and providing a community platform, where we all get to engage in these conversations. Culture is created and we can re-create it. We have the ability to shape it the way that we want.

RB: Exactly, and, honestly, from purely a business standpoint, it's been much more beneficial for me to be consistently authentic. I mean, there are hundreds of "yoga girls" out there all wanting to do the same thing, and I've been able to really separate myself from that movement of people that all do the same thing. You know, it's a gorgeous inversion on a beach with a copy and paste quote, all the tags of everything they're wearing and it's just not, at least to me, it's just not at all exciting or special at all. It all looks and reads the same. If I had gone that really commercial route, I don't think I'd have the strong and engaged community I have now. At least, I don't think it'd be as genuine as it is, for sure. I'm really happy that I followed my intuition from the start and have stayed clear on my vision.

MK: And how did it start?

RB: I never had this big picture vision or idea that I was going to do something with social media or with that account at all, actually. I was just sharing my dogs, my breakfast, and my regular day-to-day life, like most people on Instagram. And then I would sprinkle little pieces of yoga stuff in there because it was just a part of my day-to-day life. And I realized really quickly that people were interested in what I had to share about yoga. But it was never really for me about the picture, more about the wording that I connected to that picture. In fact, that's when it started to grow and really explode. Yoga is a huge part of it, but in the end it's not so much about the body for me. In fact, it was never that much about the body at all. It was about the experiences and feelings I shared in words.

MK: And yet, social media is visual. And people do make it about the body.

RB: Oh, of course, of course. Because I have an Instagram account with more than two million followers, anytime I would share anything in the beginning, I'd find it super challenging to ignore the trolls and people who would do nothing but objectify and shame me for my body. I've gotten so many hurtful comments and messages, including how I am ruining the art of yoga in addition to the standard

comments that I am "an ugly slut" or "so fat." I had to quickly decide
whether I wanted to continue down this path or not.

MK: And you clearly chose to continue.

RB: Yes, because I realized I'm on a path bigger than these comments
and that I'll face criticism and negativity no matter what I do.

MK: What continues to inspire you in this work?

RB: I have a practice that inspires me, and I have words I want to share
about that practice. But I also want to present life, all of it. I try to
balance the beauty of where I live and the joy and inspiration I derive
from my practice with my insecurities, fears, and all the shit we humans must face. I want people to feel they can find inspiration on my
page, but in a way that is accessible because it's authentic and there's
a real human behind the images versus mainstream yoga magazines
that are picture perfect fantasies of real life ...

MK: ... real life that isn't digitally altered or lit perfectly.

RB: Right, because that isn't real and can actually trigger more negativity in the long run. People can get lost in social media. Someone
very close to me has the biggest dream in life to be a Victoria's Secret
model. And I tell her, "You could be anything. Anything. You could
be president. You could be an astronaut. You could be anything you
want, and you want to be a Victoria's Secret model. Why is that?"
And she tells me, "Oh, because they have the perfect life. Everybody
loves them." She's a smart girl, but that's really her perception. It's
what she has seen her whole life; she grew up with this social media
world in a way I never did because it didn't exist at that time.

MK: Yes, the pressure has definitely increased as we've become more
and more inundated with media imagery that creates and sells "perfection" and "happiness."

RB: And I want to balance that shit out by sharing when I feel horrible or
sad. I share photos of my stomach rolls or cellulite. I want people to
know that yoga is a wonderful tool, but I don't feel like a superhuman
yoga person. I'm a regular human being, digitally unaltered, and I can
still find happiness in the face of my humanity and not-so-perfect body

and not-so-perfect life. Because yoga helps me to deal with the struggles. That's where my happiness springs from, not the fantasy.

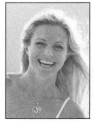 Swedish native Rachel Brathen is a *New York Times* best-selling author, serial entrepreneur, and international yoga teacher residing in Aruba. After moving to Aruba early in 2010, she started teaching yoga full-time and has spent the past seven years completely immersed in the world of yoga. With more than two million followers on social media, Brathen shares pieces of her life with the world every day and travels the globe to connect with her community through workshops, retreats, and teacher trainings.

Rachel Brathen photo by Ben Kane.

# FROM BODY ISSUES TO BODYFUL

## Pranidhi Varshney

I found yoga in the way most Americans do. I remember practicing with a video in my carpeted living room at home sometime in high school. Tae Bo was our other favorite exercise video, so my sister and I kept both in heavy rotation. If someone had told me then that yoga practice would be the cornerstone of my adult life and that teaching yoga would fulfill me in ways I dreamed of but never knew how to achieve, I would have raised an eyebrow and continued on with my uppercuts and high kicks.

This yoga video, "fat-burning yoga" I think it was, planted a small seed, which then led me to find a weekly yoga class at my gym during college. It was called "power yoga," but it was actually the full primary series of Ashtanga yoga with a few modifications. Whether this was coincidence, serendipity, or my life's calling beckoning me remains a mystery. Upon graduation, I found a local studio that offered Ashtanga and started taking a couple of classes a week. During this time of transition, the pressures of a sudden lack of community and constant professional uncertainty manifested themselves in disordered eating and body image. Yoga was part of my obsessive focus on diet and weight, along with spinning, running, and strict calorie restriction. As is the common theme, controlling my body became the stand-in for connection, purpose, and an empowered sense of where my life was headed.

Throughout this dark time, practicing yoga offered me glimpses of freedom. It allowed me to have an experience of my body outside of a scale or a mirror. Sensing that the path I was heading down was a destructive one, I consciously began to change my behaviors. Step-by-step, I cut out behaviors that I felt were no longer serving me. Eventually, one of my professional gigs took me on tour and this is when my life changed. While on tour, I had been practicing the primary series on my own a couple of times a week. During a break between cities, I signed up for a yoga retreat that happened to coincide perfectly with our vacation days. Again coincidence, serendipity, or my life's calling beckoning to me, who knows. Though this retreat was not specific to Ashtanga, I came back with the realization that I needed to practice Ashtanga yoga every day. This was not a decision I made. It was a moment of clarity and intuition. Something given to me as a boon.

So began my daily practice under the lineage that now fills my life with connection, purpose, and empowerment—the very things I had been craving as a young adult. The moment I surrendered to daily practice was the moment I began to heal. My body changed in tangible ways. First it became rounder, then heavier, then stronger, then leaner, and all the while I became a witness. Of course, the process was not so easy. The demons that come up during surrender are fierce. But disciplined practice gave me the courage to acknowledge them without giving them the power to make my decisions.

Disciplined practice allows me to accept my body in all its states—tired, weak, alive, energetic, open, in pain, and more. It allows me a profound connection to my emotional truth. It serves as a mirror on days when I feel great and days when I feel drained. It allows me to view everything as a practice—relationships, work, family. It gives me a sense of connection to something larger than myself and connects me to a community of practitioners that spans space and time.

Patanjali's *Yoga Sutras* say *yogascittavrittinirodhah*, or "yoga is the settling of the mind into silence."[1] This is an elusive goal and asana-based yoga practices give us a tangible pathway to entering this stillness. Through persistent focus on breath and body, we invite our minds to quiet naturally. We become aware of thought and behavior patterns as they rise and fall. We learn how to confront and let go of insecurities that don't serve us and find an inner strength that transcends circumstance. All this happens not through the intellect, but through a visceral experience of breath and body. The term *mindful* is often used to describe this conscious way of living, but that word doesn't do our practice justice. Our practice allows us to live fully in and through our bodies—to be *bodyful*.

## The Function of Asana

My story is not remarkable. Put simply, yoga changed my life. I share it candidly here not because of its uniqueness but because I feel that many modern yogis may have lost sight of their healing stories. We live in a time in which our relationships with our bodies have become increasingly fraught. Psychotherapist and social critic Susie Orbach says, "While we demand more rigour and have high expectations of what the fit, healthy and beautiful body can deliver for us, there is an increase in symptoms, from sexual dissatisfactions to eating problems, fear of ageing, body dysmorphia and addiction to cyber-disembodiment, which reveals how individuals struggle to make sense of the material source of their existence."[2] During a time when we need a practice that can help us integrate with our bodies, I fear that yoga may become just another expression of disorder. When practiced with correct intent, yoga gives us an inward, embodied experience of presence that is transformative. When practiced with ill intent, however, it can exacerbate existing imbalances and destroy the practitioner's well-being.

To me, the goal of yoga practice is to bring the body to health, still the mind, and come into presence and connection. This is absolutely

1. Alistair Shearer, *The Yoga Sutras of Patanjali* (New York: Bell Tower, 1982), 90.
2. Susie Orbach, *Bodies* (New York: Picador, 2009), 32.

happening in many places. Dr. Bessel van der Kolk has been instrumental in researching the positive impact yoga can have on healing trauma,[3] Matthew Sanford is revolutionizing our understanding of an awakened mind-body connection,[4] local studios around the world are sharing this sacred practice with their communities, and with yoga's increasing popularity, research is coming forth to showcase its many physical, mental, and energetic benefits.

Simultaneously, however, yoga in the public sphere seems to be a proliferation of ego-inflating behaviors. Selfies of barely clothed women and men doing fancy asana beside oceans, atop mountains, and on magazine covers dominate the public's perception of what yoga is. Yoga practice is meant to weaken the causes of suffering, one of which is our identification with the ego, or that which we think separates us from others. Perhaps some of these yogis aim simply to inspire, but it's difficult to imagine that the majority of them are not hoping to attract fame, followers, and, ultimately, bolster their own egos. Instead of practice being a space for intimate inquiry into one's own insecurities, it becomes a space for using external validation to put a Band-Aid on the pain of those insecurities. Asana then becomes part of the disease instead of the medicine, and the practice of yoga gets reduced to nothing but pretty postures done by pretty people.

## Teaching As Service

When teachers build their careers in this way, I find it particularly irresponsible. Teachers are in a position of power. Through consistent practice, they've cultivated certain abilities—physical and beyond—and they can choose how to employ these abilities. The *Yoga Sutras* warn us against overidentification with the fruits of our practice and caution us that true freedom can only be found when we relinquish our attachment to achievements. I wonder how many teachers are keeping this in mind when they proliferate an overly physical, outcome-based approach

3. Bessel van der Kolk, *The Body Keeps the Score: Brain, Mind, and Body in the Healing of Trauma* (New York: Penguin, 2014).

4. Matthew Sanford, *Waking: A Memoir of Trauma and Transcendence* (New York: Rodale, 2006).

to asana. If we continue to practice and teach in this way, not only do we impede our own progress, we pass on this attachment to our students. In this way, a generation of practitioners is being born that has little connection to the heart of the practice.

Asana is a powerful tool—one we need now more than ever. It allows us an experience of our breath and our bodies that most of us have never had. It moves energy while strengthening and comforting us. It channels the eight limbs in an accessible way. The image-based culture that many teachers are buying into these days, though, is stripping asana of these benefits and becoming exclusionary instead of inviting to many students. To these teachers, I would ask: In what ways has yoga healed you? Do you remember the sparks of self-knowledge and self-love that happened on the mat and inspired you to keep coming back? Are your choices in alignment with the answers to these questions and do they invite others to dive deeply into yoga's heart?

Teaching is not only a sacred extension of one's practice but a profound service. In contemporary yoga culture, however, conventional models of success are being applied to what should be a service-based path. If fame and financial wealth are the goals, it's no surprise that teachers feel pressured to build an image-heavy social media presence and rebrand a living, breathing, evolving practice as their own. If, however, the aim is to serve, then each action a teacher takes becomes a tool to promote inner transformation and profound contentment.

## From Transformation to Action

When the time came to build my own *shala*, Yoga Shala West in Los Angeles, these were the ideals I wanted to promote. I wanted to create the conditions for a pure-hearted, diverse, and supportive community of yogis to emerge. Through intentional design and warm reception of that design, this is the community that's emerging. At the shala, interdependence is built right into our fee structure. All of our monthly members contribute on a sliding scale. No one is turned away due to financial barriers and everyone is expected to contribute the amount that is right for them. New students are required to commit to two weeks of daily practice in order to develop discipline, and these two weeks are offered as a gift so that the student-teacher relationship can blossom without the influence of money. Our website features no images so that the experience of practice can speak for itself. Our promotional and educational videos feature a range of body types to counter the myth of the "ideal" yoga body. These and other simple design choices have attracted sincere, generous, loving students who are committed to the practice and to supporting each other.

These choices came about as a result of me asking myself strong questions during the design process. As we move forward in our journeys as teachers, studio owners, and leaders in the yoga space, we have a responsibility to ask ourselves such questions as: What can I do to keep the essence of yoga alive? How can I make this practice accessible to more people so that the circle of yoga continues to grow in richness? Am I maintaining authenticity and humility as I practice, teach, and promote?

I've designed my *shala* in response to these questions and others have found answers that are working for their chosen paths of service. Green Tree Yoga and Meditation in South Los Angeles offers all of its classes by donation, and it also offers teacher trainings on scholarship so that yogis can further serve their communities. Piedmont Yoga in Oakland recently gave up its home and transitioned to renting space from various locations so that it could continue to charge students an affordable rate and pay their teachers appropriately. Yoga thought leaders are writing articles and creating circles of sharing to deepen dialogue around these issues, and several yoga-based organizations such as Yoga Gives Back are harnessing the power of our growing community to raise resources for worthy causes. There is lots of good work being done, and there are many ways to share the fruits of yoga with more people. There is no one right answer, but we all can surely do something. As Vedic philosophy states, "One goal, many paths." If our intent is pure, it can be manifested in many ways, all useful and true.

## The Power of Authentic Community

In an increasingly polarized world, connection to one another is an essential element of our practice. Krishnamacharya urged his students to become householders and to bring yoga to other householders. Pattabhi Jois, one of Krishnamacharya's students and the founder of Ashtanga yoga as we know it, urged his students to start families. I think they both knew intuitively that the world would need this practice and that keeping it locked up in a cave would be a great disservice. Desikachar, son and lifelong student of Krishnamacharya, says, "Yoga is not merely intellectual. It is about inner transformation. And as we will see as we go on, yoga is also relationship." [5]

As more and more people come into relationship with yoga, questions of how best to share this practice naturally arise. And as an Indian-American, I sometimes feel that others look to me as an authority on what is right and wrong in that sharing. What is appropriate and what is appropriation? What is community-building and what is exploitative? For me, it comes down to authenticity and purity of intent. Yoga belongs to all dedicated students who are living their truth. I don't feel that I have any specific ownership of this practice because of my history or my brown skin, nor do I think that taking on a persona of "Indian-ness" is a prerequisite for taking practice. The modern-day conflation of yoga and Hinduism is a dangerous one. Desikachar himself says, "Yoga is not Hinduism." [6] Devotion to a connectedness that goes beyond oneself is an essential element of yoga, but Hinduism certainly is not. By mistakenly lumping these two practices into one package, we dilute yoga's essence and alienate new students who may be turned off by pseudo-spiritual trappings. It's the responsibility of each yogi to find a genuine expression of this practice—simultaneously maintaining a connection to source and a connection within.

Deepening this connection within is what allows us to fully see and connect with others. This is the work we do each day, which a good teacher can help us with. Yoga opens the door to a self-intimacy that can lead to profound healing. As we continue this work, we often effortlessly open our hearts to others. Practicing in a room with fellow human beings, breathing and moving together, we tap into a connection beyond words.

5. T.K.V. Desikachar and Hellfried Krusche, *Freud and Yoga: Two Philosophies of Mind Compared*, trans. Anne-Marie Hodges (New York: North Point Press, 2014), 23.
6. Ibid., 24.

Our inner transformation becomes collective transformation, and we're able to share growing reserves of love and compassion with our communities. If there is a goal to yoga practice, this must be it. To heal ourselves and be of service to others. For this to happen, we must stay rooted in authentic practice with correct intent. Only then can we come into a state of union.

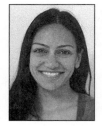

Pranidhi Varshney is the founder of Yoga Shala West, a community-supported Ashtanga yoga shala in West Los Angeles. To support yoga practice on and off the mat, she writes regularly, has released an album of Sanskrit chanting, is a Yoga Gives Back ambassador, and sits on the advisory board of the Yoga and Body Image Coalition. Through all her work, she aims to build community and touch the heart.

Author photo by Geeta Malik.

# FINDING MY YOGA HOME

## *Zubin Shroff*

My very first association with yoga was at my grandparents' house in South London. Whenever I visited, the morning would begin with my grandfather practicing yoga in the living room, usually alone. If anyone else was around, he would continue undistracted. There was no special mat or outfit or elaborate ritual—to him, yoga was as ordinary as having breakfast or going to the pub in the evening. In fact, my grandfather's daily routine was to practice yoga every morning and go to the pub every evening. He saw one of his roles as teaching me about life, so he showed me a few things about yoga to build a healthy mind and body. And in the summer when the weather was good, he would take me to the pub, which was his community. Children weren't allowed inside, so we would sit in the garden with his friends. Yoga and the pub were both equally recurring parts of our hybrid life; in the same spirit, his other passions were his perfect English lawn and his twice-daily Zoroastrian prayers.

I started to actively practice yoga when I was around twelve in a cold, drafty house in Edinburgh. We had recently moved and my mother started taking yoga classes as an opportunity to meet new friends and get fit at the same time. I would copy her when she practiced at home, making fun of her struggles to get into poses that, with a child's body, were easy for me. Wanting to emulate my grandfather, I continued to practice when my mother's busy life led to her practice slipping away. Like many things in my life, I learned from my grandfather's example, and if anything defined yoga for me, it was discipline and steadiness. Committing to this practice made me feel good, cleared my mind, and strengthened my body. It was my breath, my body, and myself. Simple, profound, and personal.

In Mumbai, my aunt and uncle and their friends had yoga classes in their homes. They studied with B. K. S. Iyengar, a popular teacher with the Mumbai Parsi community, not yet the celebrity he later became. None of them had the "yoga bodies" as understood by twenty-first–century North American yoga studios. Many of them could not touch their toes and none wore "yoga pants."

For me, yoga was my connection to family, whether in India or England; it was something done at home by ordinary Indian men and women with a vast array of body types. There were no special yoga mats or clothes and, as my family are not Hindu, no association with Hanuman or Ganesh or Siva. There was very little presence of yoga in British popular culture at the time, so there was nothing to compare my experience of yoga with.

## The Yoga Scene—Not My Scene, New York Hybridity & Searching for a Yoga Teacher

Years later, when I got my first glimpses of North American yoga, it looked and felt very alien. I was now living in New York and had worked most of my life as a photographer. In the mid 1990s, I was asked to make some images of a popular yoga studio. I entered a room of seventy to eighty sweaty people, all white, all young—Why were they sweating so much, was the air conditioner broken? I had never seen people sweat like this doing yoga. Hindu deities adorned the room, Hindu chants played in the background, and everyone greeted me with "namaste." The teachers running the studio were very generous and invited me to come and take a class, but it was too foreign to make any sense. I felt it had no connection with the yoga I understood, nor to any of the bodies I knew who practiced it. My aunts and uncles, my grandfather, their friends, they would have been completely out of place here.

A few years later, when I had a serious accident, yoga became a tool to regain my strength, reintegrate my broken body, and deal with the remaining weakness. Two years went by, and still asana that were once so easy were no longer possible. All that was left of my once active practice was the simplest breath work. At the same time, all around me, the yoga industry boomed, but I paid little attention to it. To me, the rise of this particular form that was North American yoga was just another unrealistic way India and Indian-ness were exoticised and disembodied from the actual country and from my own experiences.

But something brought me back to my practice. I realized that in striving for and achieving the conventional definition of success in my career, life had become overly complex, busy, boring. I craved balance and perspective, and I knew yoga was the tool that would help me find it. Now my practice was very different, more internal and less physical. I spent a year deeply immersing myself back into my yoga practice, but did not tell many people around me. It was not a secret; I just didn't see the connection of what I was doing to this "other" yoga that was popping up all around me. This other yoga now on billboards and in magazines, being used to sell diet pills and cars with images usually depicting the same type of person increasingly separated my understanding of yoga from this new, mainstream public face.

After this intense year of self-study, when my only yoga book, *Asana Pranayama Mudra Bandha* by Satyananda (the book my mother had originally used in the 1970s), was falling apart and bulging with post-it notes, I felt it was time to find a teacher to help me learn more. At this point, it was 2008; I still didn't own a yoga mat and I had still never been to a yoga class. In fact, the idea of practicing yoga with a room full of strangers, whatever they looked like, seemed almost indecent.

With some research, I discovered the most available way to study intensively was to do a teacher training. To my mind, becoming a yoga teacher after 200 hours of study was so unfathomable a concept, it wasn't even concerning. As I looked for trainings led by people I could identify with, I quickly understood that even if the teacher's name was

Shiva or Devi, they were probably not of South Asian origin, yet they may be wearing mala beads and bindis, quoting more Sanskrit words that any of my South Asian friends ever did. Put off by this, I considered enrolling in a training in India, but I never did well with Indian patriarchal authority, a learning style that was based on doing what you are told and not asking questions. I remember my family telling me how mean their Iyengar teachers had been and how Mr. Iyengar would sometimes kick people who weren't doing poses properly; this was not what I was looking for. Nor did I recognize myself in the growing Hindu religious expressions of yoga seen in the mass popularity of teachers like Ramdev, who used his yoga camps to promote his homophobic and Hindu fundamentalist views.

I felt stuck. My life in New York was a hybrid, contemporary one with artists, academics, and activists from Brazil, India, Iraq, and the United Kingdom all learning with North America's hyphenated and inclusive identities: Asian-American, African-American, LGBTQ, Jewish New Yorkers, all rooted in disparate traditions, creating a new hybrid one. In many ways, my own practice of yoga mirrored this—rooted in history, in family, it helped me connect with the here and now, absorbing new experiences and gaining new insight. I realized that if I were to connect with a yoga community, it would have to look the hybrid evolving one I lived in.

I did, in the end, choose a teacher training where one of the main teachers was Asian American, highly skilled and experienced, and there were a few other people of color in the class. I was planning to sit in the back, learn what I could, and go back to my own yoga practice.

Instead, I was captivated by the generosity of my teachers, Rodney Yee and Colleen Saidman, their ability to support forty other students, who in turn showed me an equal number of different ways to practice. People brought their own knowledge and experience to yoga with passion and intent. In this inclusive environment, I began to imagine the great relevance a truly diverse yoga community might have. Both yoga and South Asia have a long history of absorbing and evolving with different thoughts and cultures, all connected yet distinct. This history mirrors the vision of the United States, as a country of inclusion and experimentation, of imagining new possibilities. Perhaps yoga could help strengthen this in the face of opposing forces of isolation, alienation, and hate. I had long conversations with my fellow like-minded student (and now yoga sister) Ericka Phillips. We both imagined a radically inclusive yoga community that both reflected and helped us navigate our lives and interests.

## Spiritual Bypass, Appropriation & Exclusion

At the same time, I attended other classes that made me feel I was back in 1980s London. One where a teacher, trying to help students pronounce proper Sanskrit, suggested they wobble their heads and talk with the kind of accents I had only previously heard in racist taunts and the absurd characterizations in the *Carry On* films of sixties and seventies Britain. Other classes taught mistellings of Hindu myths and made sweeping generalizations of Indian culture.

I felt the vibrant and complex idea that is South Asian being stripped away and replaced with an exotic and ancient Indian simulacrum used to make one feel spiritual and universal and bypass any understanding or engagement with the real world we live in. It was clear that most of my South Asian friends had a great dislike for all things being presented as yoga, my international friends largely ignored it, and those involved with social justice saw it as part of the problem.

I heard black and brown people honestly saying yoga is just for white people. The truly painful part was I could see how they could think that. I saw how the yoga taught in many mainstream studios often perpetuated beauty myths and body-shamed many who did not conform with its idealized image; how complicated poses were experienced as something you failed at rather than a tool to reveal and celebrate one's own body; how *dharma* talks of "we are all one" could easily be used to ignore issues of race, gender, and sexuality that separate us and our responsibility for creating the world we live in.

Despite the increasingly problematic mainstream face, I did begin to meet people in the undercurrent—individuals and groups that were both honoring the tradition and making the practice contemporary, who saw yoga as not just a pursuit of flexibility but a way of life, as a spiritual practice that could be put into service to support just and inclusive communities. I met people who taught in halfway houses, incorporating yoga into mental health fields, teaching donation-based classes, and working with communities of color. Meeting so many committed yogis made me ask myself what my role was. What could I do to offer this practice that has been so important in my life to those who were being excluded and build a yoga community that was relevant to my life and most of the people I knew?

## California: No, We Are Not All One, Diversity, & Resistance

After I moved to the Bay Area, a chain of circumstances led to me being asked to take over the running of a well-established studio in Oakland, and I saw an opportunity. My goal was threefold: to teach yoga as a multifaceted practice that would equally include asana, meditation, *pranayama*, and self-discovery, to build a diverse community of both students and teachers, and to use the practice as a guide to skillful living and service.

Naively, I was surprised by the strength of resistance I encountered from the existing community. Diversity and inclusion are easier to talk about than practice. Whilst the studio had many talented teachers of asana, body mechanics, and breathing practices, I saw little if any interest in supporting self-exploration or accountability for one's actions and the society we live in. The social structure was not welcoming to the new teachers or students I was trying to attract. The studio felt like an island isolated from the Oakland that was walking in the streets outside, and it didn't want its sanctuary disturbed. Safe space is a popular idea in yoga studios, but what does a safe space look like? Is the aim of a safe space to protect us from facing our fears and misunderstandings or does it serve us better as a place where we are able to sit together and explore our own discomfort and responsibility—a space for honesty and for transformation? If making a space that is safe for us contributes to a lack of safety for our neighbors is this really practicing yoga?

To diversify our community, I saw it essential to bring in teachers of color, to actively invite a diverse population into our teacher trainings, and to teach in a way that they would feel included and valued. Unfortunately, the teachers of color I did attract didn't stay, as they didn't feel comfortable in the existing culture, and many of the increasingly diverse student body did not feel seen or heard by the predominantly white faculty.

What I thought would be a relatively easy transition turned into a multi-year battle that was confusing and isolating. I had hoped the change would be gradual and inclusive, assimilating the existing studio community with the new community I imagined, but this was not to be. The great fortune of resistance is that it can be used to clarify your vision and strengthen your resolve, and with the help of other teachers and students the path became clear. Eventually, I turned to my own community of teachers and supportive allies who have always been near in times of need. I had met Ericka Huggins a couple of years prior, when I interviewed her for a book I was working on, and I called on her for help. She understood my vision and, with her ever-present generosity, supported me unflinchingly and guided me through this difficult time, and I am constantly grateful for her support.

## Finding Community in Oakland

The clarity that was revealing itself was further directed by the social climate we are living in, where more and more people are awakening to the great turmoil around us: weekly videos of police brutality, of a deeply divisive political climate, and of powerful new visions provided by activists challenge our understanding of leadership and whose voices are valued. This clarity was matched by the certainty of how relevant a spiritual practice like yoga is to help us build a culture of self-care and build the supportive and skillful communities needed to lead us into change that is loving, just, and transformational. With this clarity and purpose came the strength to make big and uncomfortable changes to the structure of the studio and the support of more and more teachers and students who had the same vision.

Today, our studio is supported by a rich, loving group of friends and allies, where we teach and learn in collective groups of students and teachers. We challenge the idea of a teacher as one with ultimate authority who passes out knowledge as they wish and, instead, we try and see that at all times knowledge and moral, ethical, and spiritual authority flows between different members of the group. We challenge ourselves with honest, and sometimes uncomfortable, conversations. In this process, many of us find healing and truth, while others feel too confronted. As I continue this work, I realize that to have an honest and transformative community, we cannot all agree and some will fall away and that has to be okay.

In this yoga community that I feel so honored to be a part of, I see that as we continue to learn how to challenge our assumptions, work with conflict, and strengthen our voices, our practice together is often difficult and imperfect and constantly evolving. I see us celebrating this with a spirit of generosity, forgiveness, and inquiry. I finally feel part of a yoga community that mirrors my world outside yoga. I finally feel my own individual yoga practice has found its home.

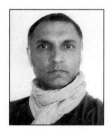

As director of Piedmont Yoga, Zubin oversees and informs the future direction of the studio. He teaches in the 200-hour and 300-hour teacher trainings and in the Integrative Yoga Therapy Teacher Trainings, as well as in Oakland public schools and in hospitals. Zubin is the author of *Conversations with Modern Yogis*, a comprehensive collection of his interviews and portraits of yoga practitioners and teachers in North America, and *The Cosmopolitans*, a collection of portraits exploring the meaning of cultural identity.

Author photo by Zubin Shroff.

# LESSONS LEARNED, LESSONS TAUGHT

## Dr. Gail Parker

Yoga saved my life. I love yoga and have practiced it all of my adult life. It has and continues to shape my consciousness, and it teaches me that my power lies in my ability to create my own destiny through awareness, intention, desire, and focus.

To set the stage, I came of age during the Black Power, Civil Rights, and Black Is Beautiful movements. Angela Davis and Nina Simone were my "sheroes." Sporting an afro, which was every bit as full as Angela's, was an outward manifestation of my commitment to dispelling the notion that there was something inherently unattractive about black people's natural appearance. Black really was powerful and beautiful and I wanted the world to know that I regarded myself, and all black women as both. What I hadn't learned yet was the power of loving myself from the inside out. Yoga taught me that. This is a story of how my consciousness evolved through body awareness.

In the late 1960s, I met a man at a college rally sponsored by the Congress of Racial Equality. Interracial dating was frowned on at the time, college students faced expulsion for it, and interracial marriage was still illegal in some states. In spite of that, or maybe even because of it, we decided, after a three-month courtship, to get married to show the world, including our parents who disapproved, that we could change the world. We married the same year the Supreme Court ruled laws on mixed-raced marriages illegal. We were both twenty and barely knew each other.

As I look back on it, our marriage was an act of political defiance more than anything else. I naively thought that this act of open rebellion could change other people's hearts and minds. I did not know at the time that the only heart and mind you can change is your own, and that you can only accomplish that through individual personal transformation, not by acting out. I learned this lesson the hard way through experience. Teaching it to others became my life's work.

My husband turned out to be a verbally, emotionally, and physically abusive man. The day we got married, and for the following year, I was the object of his abuse. His violent rages seemed to come out of nowhere. I was terrified of him and was as careful as I knew how to be not to trigger him. I walked on eggshells continuously. Nothing worked. No matter what I did the abuse continued. Why didn't I leave? Circumstance and pride. In 1967, no-fault divorce was not an option, domestic violence was not considered a crime, and blame the victim was the name of the game. To make matters worse, I was ashamed of myself for marrying someone I barely knew. I blamed myself for his abuse, and I blamed myself for taking it. So I didn't tell anyone what was going on. Instead I stayed and tried to make the best of a bad situation.

We shared a car. Both of us worked. It was my habit to pick him up from work in the evening. One afternoon I made a decision to remain at work to complete an interview I was conducting. I had no way to reach him to let him know that I would be about fifteen minutes late (there were no cell phones then). When I arrived to pick him up, he was not there. My heart sank. Instead of waiting for me, he had taken the bus home in a driving rainstorm.

I knew he would be furious by the time I arrived home, and sure enough, there he was waiting for me inside the foyer of our apartment with a leather belt in his hand. When I walked through the door, he began screaming obscenities at me and beating me with the belt. As usual, I was totally unprepared for the assault.

Afraid to defend myself, I felt victimized and helpless. But there was something different this time. I am not really certain how long the attack continued, but at some point during it, time slowed down, almost coming to a standstill. I felt as though my body was floating above the scene of this whipping, and I remember hearing a voice inside my head say as clearly as if there had been someone in the room talking to me, "You know he's crazy, but you must be crazy too for putting up with this." And then something in me literally clicked. In the instant of becoming conscious of my own insanity, I was transformed from the victim of an abusive husband into a woman who had choices. I knew then, even though I was not yet ready emotionally or financially, that I would leave the relationship.

I never said a word to him or lifted a finger to defend myself, but the most amazing thing happened. Immediately following, or maybe simultaneous to becoming aware of my own craziness for putting up with the situation coupled with my decision to leave, he stopped hitting me and screaming at me, dropped the belt, and walked away. We never once spoke of the incident, and yet he never raised his voice to me or lifted a finger to harm me in any way after that. Miraculously, it was as if he somehow sensed that he would never be able to treat me that way again, and I knew it too. Something in me had shifted.

In a moment of profound awareness, I had taken personal responsibility for my own sense of well-being. In an instant, I had changed on a deep, fundamental level. The shift in me completely changed the way I regarded myself and profoundly changed the way he interacted with me forever. Once I realized that I had choices, within months I was enrolled in graduate school, moved out of our apartment, and filed for divorce. My newfound freedom came from my awareness of myself as a worthwhile human being, deserving of all the good that life has to offer, with the power to choose the life I wanted to live. I was no longer a victim. I was free.

I didn't realize it at the time, but looking back, I now know that it was yoga, which I had been practicing for about one year when this event took place, that woke me up and ultimately saved me.

## Yoga Transforms the Body, Heart, and Mind

The same year I got married, out of curiosity, I took my first yoga class at the local art museum. There were no yoga studios at the time. My teacher, I later learned, was regarded as one of Paramahansa Yogananda's (*Autobiography of a Yogi*) foremost disciples. Without realizing it at the time, I was introduced to yoga by the teachings of a master. After my first class, I was hooked. In addition to Hatha Yoga classes, my yoga teacher also offered weekly Sunday services. He would read Paramahansa Yogananda's Sunday Service lectures and then lead a meditation practice. I practiced and studied with him for one year before my individual personal transformation became obvious to me. That was fifty years ago, and I have been practicing yoga ever since.

My experience of yoga is and always has been that yoga is an inside out job. We actually change internally before the change shows up in our lives. It doesn't change us all at once. Yoga is a transformative practice that changes us incrementally. Bit by bit, over time, it transforms the body by increasing balance and flexibility; it cultivates steadiness of mind and calms emotions in the midst of obstacles and challenges; it cultivates mental clarity and helps access intuition and the ability to listen to yourself and others at a deep and subtle level; it strengthens your capacity for self-love, fortifies your ability for self-acceptance, and emboldens your desire to be truthful and honest, not only with others, but even more importantly with your self.

The first principle of yoga is *ahimsa*, nonviolence. It teaches us to treat others with loving-kindness and to love ourselves as well. Regardless of the messages and stereotypes about body image that have been culturally communicated to us, yoga has, without fail, helped me love the skin and shape I'm in both on and off my yoga mat. Over my lifetime, I have experienced my hair as too long or too short, too curly or not curly enough, my skin color as too dark or too light, my body shape as too skinny or too curvy, my nose and lips as too thin or too full, my voice as too loud or too soft, my facial expressions as too serious or not serious enough. I'm sure there is more, but after fifty years of practicing yoga, my focus has turned away from my image and has become increasingly internal and more focused on my essence. Yoga heals bodies, minds, and hearts.

As a seventy-year-old woman, I am more focused on who I am, and less concerned with what I look like, or what others think about my looks. This is reflected in my yoga practice. Although I still practice asana five days a week, it is with more internal awareness. Additionally, it is by practicing restorative yoga a minimum of once a week that I strengthen my internal focus. I've discovered that being still brings me into alignment with my creative intelligence and an inner state of openness that supports wise actions. Over time, my asana practice has taken a back seat in importance to my meditation practice. I have always meditated twice a day, but meditation is my priority now. My growth continues.

## Transformation Is a Never-Ending Process

I kept the story of being victimized by an abusive man a secret for more than thirty years until one day a student in a class called Change the World, that I was teaching at the University of Michigan, asked if it was possible to change abusive relationships through individual personal transformation. Prior to this, I had never told anyone this story—not my parents, my brother, my current husband, or any of my closest friends. I had buried the memory of that chapter of my life and, along with it, the feelings of humiliation and shame I had felt.

In response to the student's question, I found my voice and told the story. Before I could feel regret or embarrassment about what I had shared in a very public forum, to my surprise, someone in the class said, "That is an incredibly powerful story. Thank you for sharing it."

In telling the story, I experienced another internal shift and learned an important lesson. By making myself vulnerable and sharing a story that I had secretly regarded as a sign of my own weakness, I felt the story transform from a shameful, humiliating episode in my life into a story of courage and strength. In telling the story, which was in and of itself an act of courage, once again my perspective shifted.

The fundamental change in me, by telling that story, was my willingness to lovingly and wholeheartedly embrace those parts of me that I had for years regarded as flawed. This shift in perspective forever changed how I see myself and how I relate to the world. My clients and students have benefited from this shift, as I am much better able to help them lovingly embrace their weaknesses and flaws, which paradoxically transforms them into strengths. My family and friends also benefit, as I am much less guarded and defensive, more willing to be open and vulnerable, and have a greater sense of self-esteem, all of which allows for greater intimacy and closeness.

So the upshot of what occurred for me by finally telling this story was that another pathway opened to transforming what I had internalized as a shameful experience, to be kept secret, into a story of courage and strength that I now use to instruct others, and to be a more compassionate, open, and loving person. It also released me from a long-held but deeply buried belief that I am not "good enough," which has opened many internal doors that were formerly locked away, freeing me to be more authentic, genuine, and efficacious in all that I do.

## Tell the Story

Yoga, which means to yoke or connect, has taught me something else. Whether it's an embarrassing story, a secret crush, or a family skeleton, each of us needs someone to confide in. Yet some truths seem so deep and dark we keep them hidden from everyone—our parents, our spouse, our siblings, or a best friend—hoping no one will ever find out about them.

The problem with carrying around a secret is that it can be toxic, costing you peace of mind, happiness, and even your health. Keeping secrets interferes with your ability to be yourself and to be intimate with others. Hiding parts of your personal history takes energy and is stressful. Ongoing stress poses a health problem due to increased hormone levels that cause inflammation and compromise the immune system. These are some of the reasons keeping secrets is a dangerous practice.

It doesn't matter what your secret is: hiding debt, telling or concealing a lie, secretly eating or starving, drug addiction, alcohol abuse, or covering up physical and sexual abuse. Keeping secrets is a form of dishonesty that causes harm to us physically, psychologically, and spiritually, and sometimes it causes harm to others.

Yoga teaches us that truthfulness, *satya*, is a guiding principle of our practice both on and off our yoga mat. Our yoga practice teaches us that by shining the light of awareness on the hidden places within ourselves we can safely avoid their stress-related consequences. Even though the thought of revealing a secret can seem scary, once you take that first step, it gets easier.

## Love Yourself / Change the World

I hope telling my story helps you find the courage to tell your story, whatever it may be, and to experience the loving embrace of all those with whom you share it. Yoga supports connection and intimacy to yourself and to others. It supports community. This is power. Secrecy supports denial, disconnection, isolation, and enables the continuation of abuse and other dysfunctional behaviors. This is disempowerment. Don't get it twisted. There is no shame or weakness in being abused. The shame and weakness belong to the abuser; to all those who blame the victims of abuse; and to those individuals and institutions who would have you cover it up, hide it behind closed doors, and keep abuse a secret.

Unless you are a powerless child, being victimized does not define you as a victim. As an adult, regardless of your circumstance, no matter how it looks, no matter what you may think, you always have choices. The choice is to love yourself unconditionally. Your power lies in knowing that. I discovered this through the study and practice of yoga. Whatever path you choose to follow, make sure it's a path that teaches you to love yourself from the inside out. Find your strength. Claim your power. Stand tall. Stand proud. Love yourself. Find your voice. Tell your story. Change the world.

## Takeaway

When you're preparing to be open with others about a secret you've been harboring, a good first step is to be honest with yourself. Journal, write a poem, draw a picture, or even write a song about the secret. When you feel more comfortable about sharing the secret, try role-playing what you'll say with a trusted friend before you reveal the secret directly to others. If you don't feel comfortable divulging the secret to someone you know, seek help from a professional who is obligated to maintain confidentiality.

Here are some suggestions that can help make sharing your secret a positive experience:

- Choose someone who is trustworthy, a good listener, open-minded, nonreactive, and nonjudgmental.

- Choose a place where you have sufficient privacy and a time where there are no distractions.

- Choose someone whose loyalties are not divided and who will not feel the need to tell another friend or his or her spouse what you've shared.

- Keep in mind that therapists and clergy are sworn to maintain confidentiality so long as your secret doesn't involve doing potential harm to yourself or another person.

Remember what matters most is not the secrets you're keeping. What really matters are the friends and family who still love you once you share the truth with them.

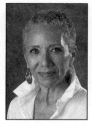

Gail Parker, PhD, E-RYT 500, is a nationally and internationally renowned media personality, educator, author, and thought leader. Her broad expertise in behavioral health and wellness include trailblazing efforts to integrate psychology, restorative yoga, and meditation as effective self-help strategies that restore emotional balance by reducing stress, anxiety, and symptoms of mild depression. She authors a blog called Taking Yoga Off Your Mat™: http://drgailparker.wordpress.com.

Author photo by Shekenia Mann.

# PART 5 MOVING INWARD & UPWARD

- How can yoga practice help you move outside your comfort zone?
- Think of at least two ways yoga can help you foster the personal and collective change you deem important.
- If you were able to call on your inner yoga renegade, what shifts would you create?
- What do you fear most but desire deeply? How can your inner yoga renegade help you?
- Who inspires you? Who are your role models?
- How can you seek out other like-minded and inspiring individuals to collaborate and commune with on your journey as an agent of change?
- What is one action, no matter how small, you can take today to create positive and meaningful change?

# CONCLUSION

## *Moving Forward*

It's true, there is no one-size-fits-all approach to the transformative journey that leads to healing and, hopefully, peace. One thing is for sure, though, and that is that yoga practice, in all it's myriad forms and styles, can be an invaluable tool. The stories in this collection affirm this truth over and over again. Often, it is yoga practice that can help someone take the first step in making positive change. Other times, yoga practice supports the journey, one that is inevitably bumpy in parts. Sometimes, it's both. And, no doubt, yoga practice can help maintain and sustain us throughout our lives.

And that is the binding thread—yoga as a healing balm for the various personal and social wounds that we, in all our diversity, possess. While yoga is by no means a cure-all or a magic elixir, it is a powerful mechanism for healing when practiced regularly and consistently. As the fearless writers share in this book, yoga usually goes hand-in-hand with one, if not several other, types of healing modalities, anything from talking therapy to time outdoors in the magnificence of nature. That's the beauty of it, while we all have a story to share, a truth to proclaim, that story is uniquely our own. While yoga should be (and can be) available to all, the role it plays in our journey is uniquely our own.

It is my deepest desire that the shared narratives in this book will allow you to gain new experiences, not just words on a page. I hope that you are exposed to newfound and unfamiliar truths with a sense of respect and gratitude for the writers sharing opinions and experiences that differ from yours, thereby expanding *your* awareness and perspective. As I stated in the introduction, it is also my great hope that you will be able to see yourself reflected and/or be able to connect to at least one, if not more, of the stories you read. And in that reflection, you feel seen and affirmed. That you are able to recognize their own truth and the value of their experiences and lived wisdom.

As *Yoga and Body Image: 25 Personal Stories About Beauty, Bravery & Loving Your Body* demonstrated, yoga can have a profound positive impact on body image distortions, an unhealthy body image, disordered eating, and, often, clinical eating disorders. This collection deepens the narrative by also focusing on how we can grow to be our best selves when we are no longer bogged down by the pain, shame, and guilt that accompanies a skewed and negative perception of ourselves and our right to take up space in the world or to simply be.

This series of stories serve as an inspiring example of how we can become active agents of change in the world when we are liberated from the incessant chatter that tries to convince us that were not good enough or not worthy. That is not to say, as many contributors noted in their essays, that yoga will switch on a light that can never grow dim. Of course, we'll continue to have challenges and recurring doubts, but yoga can serve as the conduit of energy that continues to support and ignite us. I'm quite candid when I talk about the ways yoga practice improved my self-esteem, helped move through waves of grief when my ex-boyfriend died of an overdose, supported me through years of mild depression, and improved my negative body image and disordered eating. But I am also always honest about the fact that it isn't always easy, it just becomes *easier.* And it's our job to do the work, feed the flame, and live the practice. That's when and where we become agents of change.

An agent of change can take many forms. As the writers in this book reveal, they each harnessed their power and ability to create change differently and uniquely. Whether we create changes in yoga culture to allow more people and communities to access yoga practice or stand our ground in a relationship where there has been an unhealthy dynamic or we feel compelled to work the polls, there are endless ways to become active and engaged in our lives, relationships, and communities. In the end, however, we do the work of creating positive change, everyone benefits from the distinctive gifts we have to offer. When we move toward a more inclusive, equitable, loving, and just society, we all win, and we win big.

At the beginning of this book, I also stated that it was my goal to demonstrate how the "personal is political"—how our everyday lives are not separate from the world around us. In fact, they exist in an ongoing feedback loop. Hopefully, something in this book sparked your interest to learn more about issues you were unfamiliar with previously. And maybe you'll be inspired to take action in a new way (or for the first time).

As we do the inner work to cultivate a heathy body image, improve our relationship with our body, heal ourselves, and increase our self-esteem and sense of worth, we are bolstered by the support and solidarity of others. Allow this book to offer a sense of connection to the larger whole, all of us struggling, persevering, and rising above. We all belong, we all have value, and we all deserve to be seen and heard.

I encourage you to dig deep into the resources I provide at the end. I invite you to engage in the ongoing dialogue centered on the themes in this book that continue to grow. I hope you feel compelled to work collectively with others in a way that moves you. May this book nourish and inspire you in the deepest way possible. Here's to raising consciousness and taking action. I'll be cheering you on and joining you all along the way.

The world needs you, the world needs *us*.

# RESOURCES

Are you feeling inspired? A combination of excitement and overwhelm? Well, there is certainly lots to consider and even more to learn when it comes to the intersection of yoga, body image, the diet industry, consumerism, pop culture and the media, the -isms, as well as how they relate to trauma and healing. I'm influenced and inspired by the work of countless individuals and organizations doing good work around these issues every single day. As you reflect on the stories in this collection, I'd like to share a few of the people, organizations, books, and websites that I find to be useful and thought-provoking with the intention of supporting and inspiring you long after you read the last page in this book.

While this is by no means a comprehensive list, I feel it is sufficient in providing the encouragement, knowledge, and community resources you may need now or sometime in the future. Whether you wish to deepen your understanding on your own healing journey and/or wish to support others, there's plenty here for you to explore.

## Yoga and Body Image Discussion Guides

Did you know the Yoga and Body Image Coalition website offers free downloadable discussion guides written by Dr. Beth Berila? If you're looking to dive into the stories in the first anthology, *Yoga & Body Image: 25 Stories About Beauty, Bravery and Loving Your Body,* or the stories in this volume, this guide provides thought-provoking prompts that will encourage you to examine the content from new angles as well as provide context for how to lead Yoga and Body Image group discussions.

http://yogaandbodyimage.org/discussion-guide/

## Yoga and Body Image Online Immersion

Are you interested in diving in to the themes and issues in this book with a supportive online community? Equal parts virtual book club, part consciousness-raising group, and part group coaching circle, I facilitate an interactive, live online immersion with guest experts and book contributors over eight weeks. This is offered several times throughout the year. You will be guided, supported, and prompted to explore your own narrative while, most importantly, given an opportunity to re-write that narrative.

http://ybicoalition.com/mantra

## Yoga and Body Image Coalition

Are you interested in accessing content related to the themes in this book? Do you want to support work dedicated to challenging the existing media representation of yoga and creating new and diversified imagery? Do you feel called to community? Well, check out the Yoga and Body Image Coalition (YBIC). We've been creating conscious community and media content that expands the current corporate notion of the "yoga body" and *#whatayogilookslike,* thereby inviting *every* body to the practice. A grass-roots movement rooted in social justice and equity, we've been putting our values into action since 2014.

http://ybicoalition.com/

Community is where it's at and I want to list (in alphabetical order) just a few of the countless groups and organizations offering live trainings and events, video seminars, e-courses, podcasts, compelling articles, and conferences to increase awareness, educate, and train people looking to diversify their skill set, build compassion and sensitivity as well as bolster solidarity.

# About-Face

Educating and equipping girls and women with tools to resist harmful media messages.

https://www.about-face.org

# Accessible Yoga

Trainings and conferences worldwide aimed at expanding access to the practices of yoga for people with disabilities, chronic illness, seniors, and for anyone who doesn't feel comfortable in the average studio yoga class.

http://www.accessibleyoga.org

# Adios Barbie

The one-stop body image shop for identity issues including race, size, aging, sexuality, disability, etc., since 1998.

http://www.adiosbarbie.com

# Austin Queer Yoga Collective

Decolonizing yoga and wellness through body-positivity, inclusiveness, and trauma sensitivity for the LGBTQIA+ community.

http://www.austinqueeryoga.org

# Black Girl In Om

Promoting holistic wellness and inner beauty for women of color.

http://www.blackgirlinom.com

# Black Yoga Teacher's Alliance

A professional collective and annual conference gathering aimed at community building and networking.

http://www.blackyogateachersalliance.org

# Beauty Redefined

A nonprofit working to help girls and women redefine the meaning and value of beauty in their lives.

https://beautyredefined.org

## The Body Positive

A national organization offering resources and programming to end the negative impacts of a negative body image.

http://www.thebodypositive.org

## Buddha Body Yoga

Adapting yoga poses through the use of props and providing variations on asana to increase accessibility for larger bodied people and people with injuries.

https://www.buddhabodyyoganyc.com

## Dances with Fat

Ragen Chastain, writer, speaker, ACE-certified health coach and activist on "life, liberty, and the pursuit of happiness are not size dependent."

https://danceswithfat.wordpress.com

## Decolonizing Yoga

News and resources covering queer/trans, body acceptance, and race issues and events as well as cultural appropriation and feminism as they intersect with yoga practice and yoga culture.

http://www.decolonizingyoga.com

## Embody Love Movement

Workshops, trainings, campus clubs, and e-courses focusing on beauty from the inside out to empower girls and women and contribute to meaningful change in the world.

http://embodylovemovement.org

## Health at Every Size (HAES)

A new peace movement that promotes social justice and supports people of all sizes in addressing health by adopting healthy behaviors and ditching "diet culture."

https://haescommunity.com

## Melissa Fabello

Fierce fab feminist on body image and sexuality.
http://www.melissafabello.com

## The Militant Baker

Blogger, author, speaker, and mental health professional Jes Baker helps you "lose the bullshit" and "liberate your body."
http://www.themilitantbaker.com

## Mind Body Solutions

Founded by the pioneering work of Matthew Sanford, MBS offers workshops, training, and classes. Their Opening Yoga to Everyone training program offers adaptive yoga instruction and they have trained more than 800 teachers nationally and internationally in this methodology.
http://www.mindbodysolutions.org

## Nalgona Positivity Pride

A Xicana/Brown*/Indigenous site that focuses on the intersection of eating disorders awareness, body-positivity, and decolonizing body love.
https://www.nalgonapositivitypride.com
http://nalgonapride.tumblr.com

## National Eating Disorders Association

Resources and local eating disorder support (United States only).
https://www.nationaleatingdisorders.org

## Off the Mat Into the World

In-person trainings and intensives as well as online classes dedicated to bridging yoga and activism using yoga, meditation and self-inquiry.
http://www.offthematintotheworld.org

## Proud2BMe

An online community for teens aimed at promoting positive body image and encouraging healthy attitudes about food and weight.
http://proud2bme.org

## Queering Yoga

Examining and delving into healing, self-discovery, and empowerment, Queering Yoga is a documentary about the Queer/Trans/QTPOC yoga movement.

http://queeringyoga.com

## *Race and Yoga Journal*

Exploring the intersection of yoga with whiteness, race, racialization, and liberation for all, *Race and Yoga* is the first peer-reviewed scholarly interdisciplinary journal of its kind.

http://escholarship.org/uc/crg_raceandyoga

## Red Clay Yoga

With a focus on youth and marginalized communities, Red Clay Yoga (founded by Dr. Chelsea Jackson Roberts) provides training, community engagement, restorative justice, and literacy.

http://redclayyoga.org

## South Asian American Perspectives on Yoga in America (SAAPYA)

SAAPYA is a platform and network dedicated to highlighting and uplifting the voices of yoga students and teachers across the South Asian diaspora.

https://saapya.wordpress.com

## Stonewall Yoga

A queer yoga network dedicated to inclusivity and accessibility through low pricing while raising funds for charity.

http://stonewallyogadc.net

## Trans Folx Fighting Eating Disorders

Based in Los Angeles, T-FFED is a collective of trans/gender diverse folx and allies offering trainings and supportive structures for members of marginalized communities with eating disorders.

http://www.transfolxfightingeds.org

## Trauma-Informed Yoga

A training for yoga teachers, clinicians, social workers, medical personnel, and/or individuals working with communities with trauma facilitated by Hala Khouri and/or Kyra Haglund.

http://www.traumainformedyoga.net

## Yoga Dork

On the cutting edge of yoga news and breaking stories, Yoga Dork's commentary is sprinkled with wit and wisdom.

http://yogadork.com

## Yoga for All

Live and online yoga teacher trainings educating yoga teachers and students on how to create body-positive yoga classes and spaces for people of all shapes, sizes, and abilities. Yoga for All also fosters and nurtures community engagement and support.

https://yogaforalltraining.com

## Yoga International

Dedicated to creating a cultural shift in the dominant yoga narrative, Yoga International is an online publication that provides news and commentary as well as online yoga classes, video summits, and conferences.

https://yogainternational.com

## Yoga Service Council

A collaborative community dedicated to supporting the yoga service community by offering an array of tools and projects, including their annual conference, as well as collaborative community to meet their mission.

https://yogaservicecouncil.org

# Yoga & Social Justice Collaborative

With a focus on spiritual and social justice, this collaborative offers conversation panels, events, workshops, and conferences intended to make yoga more inclusive and supportive in the name of collective liberation.
https://www.yogaandsocialjustice.com

For all my bookworms, here are some must-haves for your reading list or library. Again, this is not meant to be an exhaustive list, just a few gems I think you need to continue the journey of discovery. There's lots of smarty-pants analysis and commentary on themes related to this book, often provocative and challenging as well as deeply nourishing and enlightening.

Atkins, Dawn, ed. *Looking Queer: Body Image and Identity in Lesbian, Bisexual, Gay, and Transgender Communities*. Binghapmton, NY: Hayworth Press, 1998.

Berila, Beth, et al., eds., *Yoga, the Body, and Embodied Social Change: An Intersectional Feminist Analysis*. Lanham, MD: Lexington Press, 2016.

Butera, Robert, and Erin Byron, eds. *Llewellyn's Complete Book of Mindful Living: Awareness and Meditation Practices for Living in the Present Moment*. Woodbury, MN: Llewellyn Worldwide, 2016.

Coffin, Nancy. *Chair Yoga for Seniors: A Gentle Sequence to Get You Started*. 2013. Kindle edition.

Costin, Carolyn, and Joe Kelly, eds. *Yoga and Eating Disorders: Ancient Healing for Modern Illness*. New York: Routledge, 2016.

Eisenberg, Mindy. *Adaptive Yoga Moves Any Body*. Orange Cat Press, 2015.

Emerson, David, and Elizabeth Hopper. *Overcoming Trauma through Yoga: Reclaiming Your Body*. Berkeley, CA: North Atlantic Books, 2011.

Fries, Jonna, and Veronica Sullivan, eds. *Eating Disorders in Special Populations: Medical, Nutritional, and Psychological Treatments*. Boca Raton, FL: CRC Press/Taylor & Francis Group, 2017.

Guest-Jelley, Anna. *Curvy Yoga: Love Yourself & Your Body a Little More Each Day*. New York, NY: Sterling, 2017.

Harry, Sarah. *Fat Yoga: Yoga for All Bodies.* Sydney: New Holland, 2017.

Horton, Carol. *Yoga Ph.D.: Integrating the Life of the Mind and the Wisdom of the Body.* Chicago, IL: Kleio Books, 2012.

Horton, Carol, and Roseanne Harvey, eds. *21st Century Yoga: Culture, Politics and Practice.* Chicago, IL: Kleio Books, 2012.

Klein, Melanie, and Anna Guest-Jelley. *Yoga and Body Image: 25 Personal Stories About Beauty, Bravery & Loving Your Body.* Woodbury, MN: Llewellyn Worldwide, 2014.

Jain, Andrea R. *Selling Yoga: From Counterculture to Pop Culture.* New York: Oxford Press, 2015.

Lee, Cyndi. *May I Be Happy: A Memoir of Love, Yoga & Changing My Mind.* New York: Dutton Books, 2013.

Lipton, Laura. *Yoga Bodies: Real People, Real Stories, & the Power of Transformation.* San Francisco: Chronicle Books, 2017.

Marsh, Sarahjoy. *Hunger, Hope and Healing: A Yoga Approach to Reclaiming Your Relationship to Your Body and Food.* Boston: Shambala Publications, 2015.

Molinary, Rosie. *Beautiful You: A Daily Guide to Radical Self-Acceptance.* Berkeley, CA: Seal Press, 2010.

———. *Hijas Americanas: Beauty, Body Image, and Growing Up Latina.* Emeryville, CA: Seal Press, 2007.

Sagun, Valerie. *Big Gal Yoga: Poses and Practices to Celebrate Your Body and Empower Your Life.* Berkeley, CA: Seal Press, 2017.

Scritchfield, Rebecca. *Body Kindness: Transform Your Health from the Inside Out—And Never Say Diet Again.* New York: Workman Publishing, 2016.

Sell, Christina. *Yoga from the Inside Out.* Prescott, AZ: HOHM Press, 2003.

Simpkins, Kimber. *52 Ways to Love Your Body.* Oakland, CA: New Harbinger Press, 2016.

Smith, Dana. *YES! Yoga Has Curves.* Spiritual Essence Yoga, 2014.

Stanley, Jessamyn. *Every Body Yoga: Let Go of Fear, Get on the Mat, Love Your Body.* New York: Workman Publishing, 2017.

Tovar, Virgie. *Hot & Heavy: Fierce Fat Girls on Life, Love & Fashion.* Berkeley, CA: Seal Press, 2012.

While this is just a select sample of all the wonderful work happening right now, I hope these individuals and organizations help buoy you on your journey from here. Remember, to check out the bios and websites for all the contributors to this anthology listed at the end of their stories as well as explore the community partners officially aligned with the Yoga and Body Image Coalition listed on the "Team" page at ybicoalition.org.

# ACKNOWLEDGMENTS

I'd like to extend my heartfelt gratitude and appreciation to all the contributors in this volume who courageously shared their stories. Your words shine bright and clear and act as a beacon of light to us all.

I want to provide special acknowledgment to a few people who have been invaluable to this project. I see you, Angela Wix! Your patience and continued support has been steadfast and strong. To my soul sister, Anna Guest-Jelley, you inspire me on the daily and I am forever grateful to you for helping launch this collective storytelling process off the ground with book one and driving the conversation forward from the beginning until now. Your encouragement and trust to go it alone this round made all the difference. Your grace, ease, and kindness continue to inspire me through the rough patches.

Natalie Cummings, what would I do without you? I'm thankful for your hard work and camaraderie in extending the words from the book into the world through the Yoga and Body Image Coalition. And where would I be without Amanda Huggins? Huge thanks to Dan Ward for being the connector. Your enthusiasm, organization, and words of encouragement kept me from diving off the deep end countless times.

I want to thank my all my colleagues and allies who work tirelessly in the name of social justice and collective transformation (you know who you are and there are too many to name). I want to reserve special gratitude for those that serve (and have served) on the Yoga and Body Image Coalition leadership team with me as well as my fellow Yoga and Social Justice Conference organizers. You sustain my drive and passion while inspiring me to do better each step of the way. Thanks for all you are and all you do in the world.

I want to thank my teachers and students for their daily doses of inspiration and wisdom over the years. The well of gratitude runs deep and makes my heart sing when I think of all you have brought to my life.

Last but not least, I want to express my love and appreciation to my family and friends. I never doubt how fortunate I am to be surrounded by such supportive and encouraging people. You make it all worthwhile and I love you endlessly.

# Keep in Touch with Melanie and the Yoga and Body Image Coalition

Yoga and Body Image Coalition:

  http://ybicoalition.com

Facebook:

  https://www.facebook.com/ybicoalition

Twitter:

  http://www.twitter.com/ybicoalition

Instagram:

  http://www.instagram.com/ybicoalition

Yoga and Body Image Book:

  http://yogaandbodyimage.org

Yoga and Body Image Book on Facebook:

  https://www.facebook.com/YogaAndBodyImage

Use the following hashtags to stay engaged with us:

*#WhatAYogiLooksLike*—Engage in our effort to challenge stereotypes about who practices yoga, who "should" practice yoga, and what a "yoga body" looks like. Yoga is more than a fitness trend, yoga is a multifaceted practice available to all. YOU are *#WhatAYogiLooksLike*.

*#EveryBodyIsAYogaBody*—Join us by boldly declaring EVERY body is a yoga body. Every age. Every race and ethnicity. Every class and socioeconomic status. Every gender identity and sexual orientation. Every size, shape, height, weight, and dis/ability.